PUBLIC EDUCATION ON DIET AND CANCER

DEVELOPMENTS IN ONCOLOGY

Recent volumes

52. M. Chatel, F. Darcel and J. Pecker (eds.): *Brain Oncology.* 1987
     ISBN 0-89838-954-2
53. M.P. Hacker, Y.S. Lazo and T.R. Tritton (eds.): *Organ Directed Toxicities of Anticancer Drugs.* 1988 ISBN 0-89838-356-0
54. M. Nicolini, (ed.): *Platinum and Other Metal Coordination Compounds in Cancer Chemotherapy.* 1988 ISBN 0-89838-358-7
55. J.R. Ryan and L.O. Baker (eds.): *Recent Concepts in Sarcoma Treatment.* 1988
     ISBN 0-89838-376-5
56. M.A. Rich, J.C. Hager and D.M. Lopez (eds.): *Breast Cancer:* Scientific and Clinical Aspects. 1988 ISBN 0-89838-387-0
57. B.A. Stoll (ed.): *Women at High Risk to Breast Cancer.* 1989
     ISBN 0-89838-416-8
58. M.A. Rich, J.C. Hager and I. Keydar (eds.): *Breast Cancer:* Progress in Biology, Clinical Management and Prevention. 1989 ISBN 0-7923-0507-8
59. P.I. Reed, M. Carboni, B.J. Johnston and S. Guadagni (eds.): *New Trends in Gastric Cancer.* Background and Videosurgery. 1990 ISBN 0-7923-8917-4
60. H.K. Awwad: *Radiation Oncology: Radiobiological and Physiological Perspectives.* The Boundary-Zone btween Clinical Radiotherapy and Fundamental Radiobiology and Physiology. 1990 ISBN 0-7923-0783-6
61. J.L. Evelhoch, W. Negendank, F.A. Valeriote and L.H. Baker (eds.): *Magnetic Resonance in Experimental and Clinical Oncology.* 1990 ISBN 0-7923-0935-9
62. B.A. Stoll (ed.): *Approaches to Breast Cancer Prevention.* 1991
     ISBN 0-7923-0995-2
63. M.J. Hill and A. Giacosa (eds.): *Causation and Prevention of Human Cancer.* 1991 ISBN 0-7923-1084-5
64. J.R.W. Masters (ed.): *Human Cancer in Primary Culture.* A Handbook. 1991
     ISBN 0-7923-1088-8
65. N. Kobayashi, T. Akera and S. Mizutani (eds): *Childhood Leukemia.* Present Problems and Future Prospects. 1991 ISBN 0-7923-1138-8
66. P. Paoletti, K. Takakura, M.D. Walker, G. Butti and S. Pezzotta (eds.): *Neuro-oncology.* 1991 ISBN 0-7923-1215-5
67. K.V. Honn, L.J. Marnett, S. Nigam and T. Walden Jr (eds.): *Eicosanoids and other Bioactive Lipids in Cancer and Radiation Injury.* 1991 ISBN 0-7923-1303-8
68. F.A. Valeriote, T.H. Corbett and L.H. Baker (eds.): *Cytotoxic Anticancer Drugs.* Models and Concepts for Drug Discovery and Development. 1992 ISBN 0-7923-1629-0
69. L. Dogliotti, A. Sapino and G. Bussolati (eds.): *Breast Cancer.* Biological and Clinical Progress. 1992 ISBN 0-7923-1655-X
70. E. Benito, A. Giacosa and M.J. Hill (eds.): *Public Education on Diet and Cancer.* 1992 ISBN 0-7923-8997-2

PUBLIC EDUCATION ON DIET AND CANCER

Proceedings of the 9th Annual Symposium of the European Organization for Cooperation in Cancer Prevention Studies (ECP), Madrid, Spain, October 17–19, 1991

edited by

Dr E BENITO
Unitat d'epidemiologia i Registre del Cancer del Mallorca
Misericordia 2
E-07012 Palma de Mallorca
Spain

Dr A GIACOSA
National Institute for Cancer Research
Viale Benedetto XV, 10
I-16132 Genova
Italy

Dr MJ HILL
European Cancer Prevention
PO Box 1199
Andover
Hants. SP10 1YN
UK

KLUWER ACADEMIC PUBLISHERS
DORDRECHT / BOSTON / LONDON

Distributors

for the United States and Canada: Kluwer Academic Publishers, PO Box 358, Accord Station, Hingham, MA 02018-0358, USA
for all other countries: Kluwer Academic Publishers Group, Distribution Center, PO Box 322, 3300 AH Dordrecht, The Netherlands

Library of Congress Cataloging-in-Publication Data

European Organization for Cooperation in Cancer Prevention Studies.
    Symposium (9th : 1991 : Madrid, Spain)
        Public education on diet and cancer : proceedings of the 9th Annual Symposium
    of the European Organization for Cooperation in Cancer Prevention Studies (ECP),
    Madrid, Spain, October 17–19, 1991 / edited by E. Benito, A. Giacosa, M.J. Hill.
        p.   cm. — (Developments in oncology.)
    Includes bibliographical references and index.
    ISBN 0-7923-8997-2
        1. Cancer—Nutritional aspects—Congresses. 2. Cancer—Prevention—Congresses.
    3. Health education—Congresses. 4. Cancer—Diet therapy—Congresses.
    I. Benito, E. II. Giacosa, A. III. Hill, M.J. IV. Title. Series.
        [DNLM: 1. Diet—adverse effects—congresses. 2. Health Education—congresses.
    3. Neoplasms—etiology—congresses. 4. Neoplasms—prevention & control—
    congresses.   W1 DE998N v. 70 / QZ 202 E89P 1991]
    RC268.45E87   1991
    616.99′405—dc20
    DNLM/DLC
    for Library of Congress   92-13419
                                                            CIP

British Library Cataloguing in Publication Data

A catalogue record for this book is available from the British Library

ISBN 0-7923-8997-2

Copyright

Published in the United Kingdom by Kluwer Academic Publishers,
PO Box 55, Lancaster, UK.

Kluwer Academic Publishers BV incorporates the publishing programmes of
D. Reidel, Martinus Nijhoff, Dr W. Junk and MTP Press.

Lasertypeset by Martin Lister Publishing Services, Bolton-le-Sands, Carnforth, Lancs.

Printed and bound in Great Britain by Billing and Sons Ltd., Worcester.

Contents

Foreword

The European Cancer Prevention Organization (ECP) was established in 1981 with the objective of developing studies of the aetiology and prevention of cancer through concerted-action European collaborative studies. It achieves this through the organization of annual symposia, the organization of workshops on subjects of topical interest and the organization of research projects.

The annual symposia have all been on themes of high priority for cancer prevention; namely Tobacco and Cancer (1983), Hormones and Sexual Factors in Human Cancer Aetiology (1984), Diet and Human Carcinogenesis (1985), Concepts and Theories in Carcinogenesis (1986), Causation and Prevention of Colorectal Cancer (1987), Gastric Carcinogenesis (1988), Breast, Ovarian and Endometrial Cancer: Aetiological and Epidemiological Relationships (1989) and Causation and Prevention of Human Cancer (1990). At the time of the 1985 symposium a workshop was organized in conjunction with IUNS to formulate a set of dietary guidelines for the prevention of human cancer. Those guidelines were published in *Nutrition and Cancer*, but since then there has been a massive increase in information on diet and cancer and so it was decided that in 1991 we would again have a symposium and an associated workshop on public education on diet and cancer. The symposium was structured into a number of sections, the first of which included a review of the various sets of published guidelines together with general background papers on dietary carcinogens, anticarcinogens (particularly the vitamins) and the value of animal models in studying diet and human cancer. The second included updates on diet in relation to major sites of carcinogenesis and on the role of specific aspects of the diet (e.g. fat, alcohol, total energy, fibre). The third session was on the Mediterranean diet whilst the final section was on aspects of the implementation of guidelines (e.g. ethical issues, the likely benefits of particular dietary changes etc). These papers were precirculated to the workshop members who then used the information to determine whether particular guidelines from 1985 needed to be modified, abandoned, reinforced, or remain unchanged. Some general conclusions are discussed in the final chapter of this book.

The whole exercise was financially supported by the Spanish League against Cancer and by the Spanish Ministry of Health to whom we would like to express our grateful thanks. We are also indebted to Theresa Gallagher who was responsible for precirculation of the papers to the workshop participants and for preparation of the papers in diskette form for the publication of this book, and to Mme Chantal Cattoir and Marie-Christine Gueurr for their hard work in the organization and administration of the meeting.

The 1992 symposium will be on precancerous lesion of the digestive tract and will be held in San Remo, Italy, on 5–7 November.

List of Contributors

Dr E Benito
Unitat d'Epidemilologia i Registre del Cancer de Mallorca, Misericordia 2, E-07012 Palma de Mallorca, Spain

Professor J Faivre
Registre des Tumeurs Digestives, Faculté de Médicine, 7 Boulevarde Jeanne d'Arc, F-21033 Dijon, France

Dr S Franceschi, Epidemiology Unit, Aviano Cancer Center, Via Pedemontana Occ, 33081 Aviano (PN), Italy

Dr A Giacosa
Instituto Scientifico Tumori, Viale Benedetto XV, 10, 16132 Genova, Italy

Dr MJ Hill
European Cancer Prevention, PO Box 1199, Andover, Hants SP10 1YN, UK

Dr PA Judd
Department of Nutrition and Dietetics, King's College (Kensington), Campden Hill Road, London W8 7AH, UK

Dr FJ Kok
CIVO-TNO, PO Box 360, NL-3700 AJ Zeist, The Netherlands

Dr AR Leeds
Department of Nutrition, Kings College (Kensington), Campden Hill Road, London W8 7AH, UK

Dr WK Lutz
Institute of Toxicology, Swiss Federal Institute of Technology and University of Zurich, Schorenstrasse 16, CH-8803 Schwerzenbach bei Zurich, Switzerland

Dr A Maskens
Avenue Lambeau 62, 1200-Brussels, Belgium

Dr PI Reed
Lady Sobell Gastrointestinal Unit, Wexham Park Hospital, Slough, Berks SL2
4HL, UK

Dr EB Thorling
Danish Cancer Society, Department of Nutrition and Cancer, Norrebrogade 44,
DK-8000 Aarhus C, Denmark

Dr A Trichopoulou
University of Athens, School of Medicine, Department of Hygiene and
Epidemiology, GR-111527 Athens, Greece

Professor G Varela
Department of Nutrition, School of Pharmacy, Universidad Complutense,
Ciudad Universitaria, 28040 Madrid, Spain

Dr C La Vecchia
Instituto di Ricerche Farmacologiche, "Mario Negri", Via Eritrea 62, 20157
Milano, Italy

Dr HCW de Vet
Department of Epidemiology and Biostatistics, PO Box 616, 6200 MD
Maastricht, The Netherlands

Dr F de Waard
Preventicon, Radboudkwartier 261, NL-3511 CK Utrecht, The Netherlands

PART ONE
GENERAL BACKGROUND

Chapter 1

Overview of Dietary Recommendations on Diet and Cancer

E BENITO

Unitat D'Epidemiologia I Registre del Cancer de Mallorca
Misericordia 2, 07012 Ciutat de Mallorca, Spain

Introduction

The factors that determine the selection of the food we eat are not very well defined. However, as a starting point, we can assume that from the very beginning human food selection relied mainly on the food availability provided by the natural ecologic system and also on biological and socio-cultural factors represented in Figure 1.

Amongst the cultural determinants, we would include the food information represented in the past by taboos, beliefs and recommendations (usually prohibitions) set down by the various religions. These influences still play an important role in several underdeveloped regions of the world.

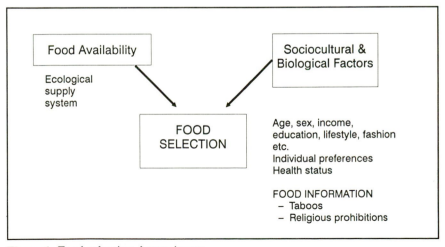

Figure 1 Food selection determinants

3

Since the beginning of the 19th century in Europe and other developed Western countries a dramatic change has happened with industrialization, urbanization, technological and economic development, leading to new forms of food production, processing and distribution. These new developments have replaced the natural ecological influences that determined our food choices and nutritional patterns for thousands of years.

The level of civilization that produced these important changes in our style of life and dietary patterns, has been associated with an increase of new health problems such as obesity, diabetes, cardiovascular diseases and cancer, nowadays recognized as characteristic diseases of our affluent societies.

In addition to the changes produced in food availability, modifications of cultural values and an increasing amount of food information are important determinants of our current food choices. From one side, former taboos have been substituted by new ones, for example, those derived from the "natural food" industry.

Besides this, an enormous amount of scientific data on diet and health has appeared in recent years, providing a new source of useful information to influence food selection in favour of a healthy diet.

The aim of this overview is to indicate the rational frame on which dietary recommendations are based, and on the other hand, to review the current available guidelines for cancer prevention and the process of their

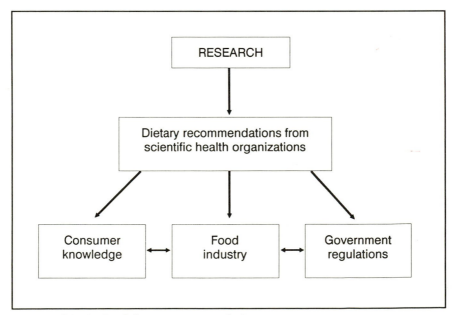

Figure 2 Ideal role of dietary recommendations

elaboration to help us to try to improve the efficacy of our own future recommendations.

Rationale of Dietary Recommendations

Following the suggested scheme, in which information is one of the possible determinants of food selection (although probably not the most important) we could consider that in an ideal situation such as the one represented by Figure 2, dietary recommendations based on scientific knowledge and addressed to the elements of the production, distribution and consumption, could play an important role on prevention of diseases associated with food consumption.

How can we justify somebody becoming an advisor to other human beings on eating, which is, for people living in developed countries, one of the most frequent and pleasant of human activities? What are the reasons that justify the interference of scientists in this field of public health?

Although all these aspects will be developed later on by other authors during the Symposium, before considering the specific dietary guidelines we should briefly identify at least three important assumptions on which public health recommendations rely (summarized in Figure 3). Firstly, we assume that the available scientific evidence on the relationship between

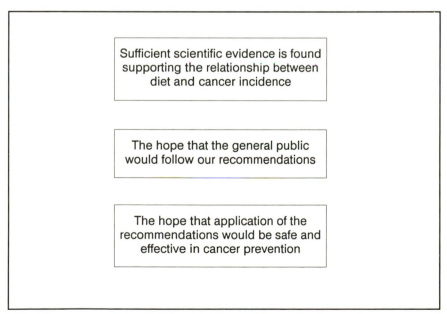

Figure 3 Rationale for dietary recommendations to the public

diet and cancer is sufficient to enable us to give advice on what, we presume, is a healthy diet. Secondly, having issued the recommendations, we hope that the people to whom these recommendations have been made will follow our advice; this is by no means certain. Last but not least, we also assume that the recommendations applied to the community would, in turn, be safe from other health hazards and effective in cancer prevention. Each of these assumptions may have important criticisms, which, as already indicated, will be discussed in greater detail later on.

Additional difficulties exist in the application of the recommendations and these can be classified into four groups:

(1) Individual variation of nutritional requirements within the population,

(2) Food choice determinants and eating behaviour,

(3) The complexity of the factors influencing food supply and,

(4) Lack of coordination between the different sectors issuing dietary guidelines.

Overview of Dietary Recommendations

Nowadays the recommendations are designed to restrain the degenerative diseases which plague the affluent western countries. In the past the nutrient deficiency diseases were important in these areas during the earlier part of this century, and these are still the major health problems in undeveloped countries. In order to combat these nutritional deficiency diseases, dietary requirements were estimated in the different countries; these usually varied depending on age and sex. These were the first dietary recommendations based on scientific knowledge.

More recently, the emerging problem of chronic diseases and their association with specific food consumption patterns resulted in a statement, produced in 1957 by the American Heart Association; this contained the first dietary recommendations for prevention of heart diseases.

In Europe, the first statements related to diet and chronic diseases were the recommendations of the Royal Norwegian Ministry of Agriculture issued in 1975, with four goals: reduce dietary fat, increase consumption of starchy foods, reduce sugar, and substitute polyunsaturated fats for saturated fats. Subsequent reports on diet and health have been developed by different institutions in almost every developed country. Some are aimed at preventing chronic diseases in general while others are specifically focused on heart disease or on cancer.

A comparison of the various sets of recommendations is not easy because of the differences in the objectives, as well as in the target

population, the presentation, and the characteristics of the countries in which they were developed. Nevertheless, in spite of these differences there is an important consensus in their contents that could be summarized in the following statements:

- Reduce dietary fat consumption

- Reduce sugar consumption

- Limit the consumption of salt

- Limit the consumption of alcohol

- Increase consumption of fibre/starch

- Increase consumption of vegetables/fruit and cereals

- Avoid overweight/maintain adequate energy balance

Other recommendations such as reduction in the consumption of cholesterol and of animal proteins, increase in the consumption of fish, take no more than three meals a day, are also often cited.

When focusing on dietary recommendations dedicated to cancer prevention, the overview becomes easier. The first such document was the "Statement on Diet, Nutrition and Cancer", issued in 1979 by the National Cancer Institute. A small number of similar statements has followed, five of which have been selected for this review and are summarized in Table 1. Amongst these five there are important similarities as shown in Table 2. The five sets of guidelines are in complete agreement in advising high consumption of vegetables and fruits and a moderate alcohol consumption. The other four recommendations referring to the consumption of salt, fibre/starch, fat, and the maintenance of body weight avoiding obesity, are also present in four out of the five sets of recommendations. The most

Table 1 Selected dietary recommendation for cancer prevention

Institution/Area	Year	Title
NCI (USA)	1979	Statement on Diet, Nutrition and Cancer
NAS (USA)	1982	Diet Nutrition and Cancer
ECP/IUNS (Europe)	1985	Dietary Recommendations to the Public
ACS (USA)	1985	Nutrition, Common sense and Cancer
NCI (USA)	1987	NCI Dietary Guidelines ✓
Dept Health (UK)	1990	Diet and Cancer

Table 2 Summary of the recommendations* on diet and cancer

Statement	No of Sets
• Increase consumption of fruit and vegetables	5/5
• Moderation in alcohol consumption	5/5
• Avoid obesity/maintain desirable body weight	4/5
• Reduce fat intake	4/5
• Reduce salt and salty foods	4/5
• Increase consumption of fibre-rich foods/ complex carbohydrates	4/5

* From the five later sets of guidelines listed in Table 1

Table 3 Statements on dietary fat consumption

1. Reduce fat intake to 30% of total calories (*NAS, 1982*)

2. Cut down total fat intake (*ACS, 1985*)

3. Decrease intake of saturated and unsaturated fat in countries where on average fat constitutes more than 30% of total food energy (*ECP/IUNS, 1985*)

4. Reduce fat intake <30% calories (*NCI, 1987*)

5. No conclusive evidence which relates fat consumption with cancer. Maintain total fat and saturated fat below 35% and 15% of calories as recommended for prevention of heart diseases (*Britain, 1990*)

important differences between these sets of guidelines are more related to their presentation than to their content; for example, Table 3 shows the different statements on fat consumption of these five sets of recommendations.

From this table we can draw various conclusions. There is no complete agreement on the degree of evidence relating to fat consumption and cancer incidence. Differences in the interpretation of scientific evidences and the degree of confidence in the studies are the causes of this disagreement (which is also repeated in other items). In spite of this, there is a consensus on reducing fat consumption below a certain level of total energy intake (usually indicated as 30%) which is also valid in the prevention of other problems such as heart disease. The ECP/IUNS recommendation on fat was unique in that the guideline for decreased fat intake was limited to those countries with a high initial intake. This idea of "targeting" recommendations will be referred to again later in this presentation.

What can be concluded is that these statements are not directly useful for public health purposes. The recommended reduction of fat consumption to below 30% of total caloric intake is unachievable for the average

person (and often even for nutrition experts) because consumers do not have the necessary food composition data when making their food choices.

This stresses the need to identify and separate two different categories of statements dedicated to reducing the risk of developing chronic degenerative diseases. These are: statements on *dietary goals* and those on *dietary guidelines*. This distinction was first suggested in the 4th European Nutrition Conference held in Amsterdam in 1983.

The dietary goals are in the form of a national target, usually expressed quantitatively (in grams, average, etc), and identify with the optimal proportions of the different nutrients in the ideal diet. In other words, dietary goals try to answer the question: What is the composition of a healthy diet?

On the other hand, the dietary guidelines should be useful indications directed to the public and therefore understandable by them. They should be expressed in terms of food groups or items, quantitated in terms of servings etc, and designed to aid people in their choice of foods and enable them to achieve the aforementioned dietary goals. In this case the guidelines try to answer the question: What should we eat to stay healthy?

Strategies in the Elaboration and Implementation of Recommendations

The distinction between these two categories of dietary recommendations shows the necessity of implanting two separate steps in their elaboration and implementation. The first step is evaluating the scientific evidence in order to establish a healthy diet. For some authors, this is a role that scientific researchers should be restricted to. The second step would be to establish practical recommendations directed to the components of the network of food production, processing and consumption, allowing for a food choice adapted to a healthy diet. This phase as part of the Public Health Policy, should be dealt with by dieticians, nutritionists and experts in the media.

The development of recommendations can vary depending on several factors, however there are some recent experiences which because of their successful outcome can be considered as possible patterns. One example is the "Nutrition Recommendations" elaborated by the Department of National Health and Welfare of Canada and published in March 1990.

The process pursued up to the publication of the recommendations was the following:

(a) Two committees were established to cover each step, namely the SRC (Scientific Review Committee) to formulate the recommendations, and the CIC (Communications Implementation Committee) dedicated to the implementation of the recommendations.

(b)   The Scientific Committee named two sub-committees formed by experts in cancer and heart diseases, and who independently elaborated recommendations directed to reducing the risk of these diseases and which were finally incorporated into more general ones. The "Nutritional Recommendations" for scientific and professional use were edited following 22 months of work during which 10 committee members assisted by 9 consultants and 56 reviewers met 21 times.

(c)   These recommendations were then translated by the Communications Implementation Committee in "Canada's Guidelines for Healthy Eating" directed to consumers, and who also elaborated more than 100 messages for different audiences (e.g. Health Departments of Official Organizations at various levels (national, autonomic, municipal, etc), Professional Organizations of nutrition and health, the food industry etc).

It is interesting to observe that the application of these recommendations is based not only on the work of the Scientific Committee, but also on the dietary habits of the population and a study of the network through which the public receives health information. If the objective of the implementation of the recommendations is to achieve a high participation by the "target population" it is surely important to take into account the characteristics of those to whom it is directed. The message would probably differ if directed to the whole population rather than to selected groups as has been suggested. It should also vary according to the alimentary habits of the population. There is evidence that a reduction in the consumption of fats can have varying consequences on the health of the population according to the composition of the fats eaten. In addition the average of consumption of some foods included in the recommendations differs amongst European Countries. In Figure 4 we observe that the energy derived from vegetables and fruit in each European country is more important in the Mediterranean ones. In consequence general statements such as "Increase your daily consumption of vegetables and fruit", would produce different results in the different countries. It can be concluded that food recommendations should take into account the food consumption patterns of each country. It is also evident that the message should be consistent with other health recommendations, understandable, easy to carry out in the normal way of life, and should stress the positive aspects of a healthy diet avoiding restrictive guidelines, and possible public concern.

The Canadian pattern which separates two important steps in the construction and implementation of the recommendations that integrate

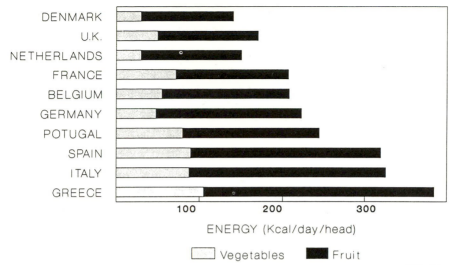

Figure 4 Energy derived from fruit and vegetables in European countries, 1979–81.
Source: Food Balance Sheets, FAO

scientific knowledge about the chronic degenerative diseases and which, at the same time, takes advantage of the distribution network of health information (bearing in mind the population to whom it is addressed) seems to be the best elaborated to date.

All this is not easy when the scientific evidence that supports this advice can be questioned and when no guarantee exists that the suggested dietary modifications will in fact reduce the risk of disease. In consequence some scientists would say that we do not know enough to be able to make good recommendations. In contrast, others would say that heart disease, diabetes, hypertension and cancer certainly cause death, and so it is our obligation to keep the public informed of our current state of knowledge and offer them the possibility of a healthy diet.

To sum up we would suggest that when elaborating future recommendations, we should take into account the basic concepts on which a healthy diet is founded namely: VARIETY, MODERATION and BALANCE. *Variety* in the institutions and professionals that take part in the elaboration of these guidelines; *moderation* in the statements directed towards a wide public, and sometimes based on controversial evidences; and *balance*, avoiding possible undesirable effects on other diseases, or any increasing of public concern about food and disease.

Finally, we should not forget that our recommendations aimed at promoting health should never set aside one of its main aspects, which is enjoyment of life. Therefore dietary recommendations should be compatible with the pleasure of enjoying food.

Acknowledgements

Thanks to Richard Dawson for editorial assistance and Nicki Smith for realisation of the manuscript.

References

American Cancer Society (1985). Nutrition, common sense and cancer. New York: American Cancer Society Inc (No 2096-LE).

Berger S (1987). The implementation of dietary guidelines: Ways and difficulties. *Am J Clin Nutr* **45:** 1382–1389.

Bingham S (1990). Diet and cancer. London: Health Education Authority.

Bruce APE (1987). The implementation of dietary guidelines. *Am J Clin Nutr* **45:** 1378–1382.

Butrum RR, Clifford CK, Lanza E (1988). NCI dietary guidelines: Rationale. *Am J Clin Nutr* **48:** 888–895.

Committee on Diet Nutrition and Cancer, Assembly of Life Sciences (1982). Diet, Nutrition and Cancer. Washington DC: National Academy Press.

De Vet HCW, Van Leeuwen FE (1986). Dietary guidelines for cancer prevention: The etiology of a confused debate. *Nutr Cancer* **8(4):** 223–229.

Dietary Guidelines Advisory Committee (1991). Report of Dietary Guidelines Advisory Committee on the Dietary Guidelines for American, 1990. United States Department of Agriculture.

Gibney MJ (1990). Dietary guidelines: A critical appraisal. *J Human Nutrition and Dietetics* **3:** 245–254.

James WPT, Ferro-Luzzi A, Isaksson B, Szostak WB (1988). Healthy nutrition: Preventing nutrition-related diseases in Europe. Copenhagen: WHO Regional Publications, European Series, No 24.

Joint ECP-IUNS Workshop (1985). Consensus Statement on Provisional Dietary Guidelines. In: Joossens JV, Hill MJ, Geboers J, eds. Diet and Human Carcinogenesis – ECP Symposium/2. Amsterdam: Elsevier Science Publishers BV, 341–342.

McNutt K (1980). Dietary advice to the public: 1957–1980. *Nutr Rev* **38(10):** 353–360.

Murray TK (1990). Nutrition recommendations. *J Can Diet Assoc* **51(3):** 391–393.

Palmer S (1983). Diet, nutrition and cancer: The future of dietary policy. *Cancer Res* **43:** 2509–2514.

Trichopoulou A, Vassilakou T (1990). Recommended dietary intakes in the European community member states: An overview. *Eur J Clin Nutr* **44:** 51–126.

Truswell AS (1987). Evolution of dietary recommendations, goals and guidelines. *Am J Clin Nutr* **45:** 1060–1072.

Woolcott DM (1990). Canada's guidelines for healthy eating: Strategies for communicating and implementing nutrition recommendations. *J Can Diet Assoc* **51(3):** 396–399.

CHAPTER 2

Carcinogens and Mutagens in the Diet

WK LUTZ[1], J SCHLATTER[2]

[1] *Institute of Toxicology*
   Swiss Federal Institute of Technology and
   University of Zurich
[2] *Toxicology Section, Division of Food Science*
   Swiss Federal Office of Public Health, CH-8603 Schwerzenbach
   Switzerland

Introduction

Diet and Cancer

Doll and Peto (1981), in their review on 'Quantitative Estimates of Avoidable Risks of Cancer' state that "it may be possible to reduce US cancer death rates by practicable dietary means by as much as 35%". This reduction results from a 90% reduction of deaths from stomach and large bowel cancer and a 50% reduction of cancer of the endometrium, gall-bladder, pancreas and breast. The degree of uncertainty in this estimate is expected to be large, however, so that values between 10% and 70% are considered possible. The authors also indicate that "there is still no precise and reliable evidence as to exactly what dietary changes would be of major importance".

Cancer is the cause of death in about one quarter of the population in Switzerland. If it is assumed that one third of this is due to the diet, about one twelfth of all deaths should be attributable to avoidable dietary carcinogens (80,000 per 1 million). In this paper, we attempt to quantify the cancer risk associated with a number of known dietary carcinogens on the basis of estimates of dose and carcinogenic potency, in order to address the question about the most important individual dietary cancer risk factors.

13

Risk = Dose x Potency

Ames and co-workers (1987) ranked possible carcinogenic hazards on the basis of human exposure estimates and carcinogenic potency in rodents (HERP-Index). They concluded for the diet that carcinogenic hazards from current levels of pesticide residues or water pollution are likely to be of minimal concern relative to the background levels of natural substances. Perera and Boffetta (1988) considered this approach inappropriate. They criticised the fact that the results were influenced by the selection of chemicals dictated by the nature and availability of both exposure and rodent potency data. In addition, they pointed out that the exposure data should have a uniform and consistent basis, such as average daily dose levels.

Our approach is based on average daily intake estimates for Switzerland, mainly from two reviews (Stähelin *et al.*, 1991; Aeschbacher, 1991). Large individual differences in exposure are mentioned for well-documented situations. In several cases, the data base for human exposure via food was poor and personal estimates had to be made. The same is true for the estimation of average carcinogenic potencies for classes of carcinogens (such as the nitroso compounds, aromatic amines, or polynuclear aromatic hydrocarbons). Whenever available, epidemiological data were taken (aflatoxin, alcohol, arsenic, benzene). In the majority of cases, however, experimental data had to be used.

For our estimations, the following assumptions were made:

1. The cancer risk is approximated by the mathematical products of dose $\times$ potency. The unit used is ng/kg bw per day. Tabulations of tumourigenic potencies have been compiled by Gold *et al.* (1984; 1986; 1987) as TD_{50}-values. The TD_{50} represents the daily dose per kg body weight which resulted in a 50% tumour incidence within 2 years. The published values were used without further evaluation.

2. Extrapolation to low dose is assumed to be linear. Nonlinearities are taken into account where the respective evidence is available.

    Example: The carcinogenic potency (TD_{50}) of ethyl carbamate (urethane) is 10 mg/kg bw per day, i.e. 10^7 ng/kg per day. The average daily intake in humans who do not consume alcoholic beverages is 20 ng/kg bw per day. This daily dose is 500,000 times lower than the dose which results in a 50% cancer incidence. Therefore, the cancer risk from ethyl carbamate in Switzerland for people who drink no alcoholic beverages is estimated to be 1 in 1 million.

Unlike with the reports by Ames *et al.* (1987) or by Perera and Boffetta (1988), our analysis allows us to sum up the single risk factors and to compare the result with the postulated number of diet-related cancer deaths. Uncertainties clearly associated with our estimate should disappear with new data becoming available.

Mutagenic Dietary Carcinogens

Table 1 lists a number of dietary carcinogens which have been shown to be mutagenic in one or more tests. The first column gives an estimate of the exposure situation in Switzerland, the second column describes the carcinogenic potency, and the third column represents the cancer risk expressed as the number of expected cases per one million lives. The reference given in the last column refers to the source of information on exposure data.

The calculated risk values span about 5 orders of magnitude and most are extremely low in view of the 80,000 cases per 10^6 which should be attributable to dietary carcinogens.

High Risk Factors

Arsenic stands out as the highest single risk factor. The ten-fold span is due to individual dietary habits with respect to the consumption of fish. The carcinogenic potency of arsenic was derived from epidemiological data (Becher and Wahrendorf, 1990). The risk values given in the Table probably represent upper limits because the dose-response relationship is unlikely to be linear for metal ion-induced carcinogenicity.

Relatively high risk factors (up to 100 cancer cases per one million lives) are derived from nitroso compounds (NOC) and aromatic amines. The average carcinogenic potency used was near the upper limit of the range. With respect to NOC exposure, this estimate does not include endogenous formation.

The formation of aromatic amines, polycyclic aromatic hydrocarbons (PAH; see below) and, in part, of NOC is largely dependent on high temperatures. This fact has to be taken into account for recommendations.

Intermediate Risk Factors

Intermediate risk factors (around 10 cases per 1 million lives) are found with other well-known classes of carcinogens, such as polycyclic aromatic hydrocarbons (PAH).

The carcinogenic metal cadmium and fungal toxins such as aflatoxin B_1, ochratoxin A or zearalenone are also intermediate risk factors. However, the exposure to fungal toxins is highly variable and largely dependent on individual nutrition habits. For instance, frequent consumption of peanuts or figs could increase the exposure to aflatoxins.

For ethyl carbamate (urethane), the risk level is largely dependent on the consumption of alcoholic beverages. While people who do not drink alcohol are at low risk, wine drinkers are in an intermediate position and regular consumption of stone-fruit brandies can represent a high risk, in comparison with most other dietary carcinogens.

Low Risk Factors

Contamination of food with benzene is thought to be primarily the result of a general contamination of the air. On this basis, the risk in Switzerland is expected to be low.

Tetrachloroethylene (PER) was formerly used for fat extraction in the food industry. These days, exposure from the diet has markedly decreased.

Negligible Risk Factors

Many carcinogens which produce headlines in the media are responsible only for a negligible dietary cancer risk. This is true for environmental contaminants (chlorinated ethylenes) or substances that migrate from packaging material (vinyl chloride or styrene) as well as for residues of veterinary drugs (dimetridazol).

The top risk apparently posed by formaldehyde (on the order of 1,000 cases per 1 million) cannot be taken at face value. This value is the result of a carcinogenic potency derived from an inhalation bioassay which showed a strongly nonlinear dose-response relationship and severe cytotoxicity in the target tissue (nasal cavities). In addition, endogenous generation of formaldehyde, for instance by oxidative demethylation reactions in cholesterol biosynthesis, is much larger than dietary formaldehyde exposure. Therefore, if low-level exposure to formaldehyde represented a substantial risk, an even larger risk would have to be attributed to unavoidable endogenous formaldehyde production.

Summary for Mutagenic Dietary Carcinogens

If we add up all the numbers collected for our selection of mutagenic dietary carcinogens we end up with only a few hundred cases per 1 million. This is far away from the alleged number of diet-related cancer deaths (80,000 per 1 million). What are the reasons for the discrepancy?

Table 1 Mutagenic dietary carcinogens – risk estimation based on daily intake and daily dose resulting in 50% tumour incidence (TD$_{50}$)

Compound	Human intake [ng/kg bw/d]	TD$_{50}$[a] [ng/kg bw/d]	Risk [cases per 10^6]	Ref[b]
Arsenic	150–500	Epi: $2-5\times10^5$	150–1200	2
Nitroso compounds, volatile	12	10^5	60	1,3
Nitroso compound, nonvolatile	150	10^6	75	
Heterocyclic aromatic amines	1.5×10^3	5×10^6-5×10^7	15–150	2
Polycyclic aromatic hydrocarbons [BaP$_{eq}$]	130–270	10^7	6–14	2,10[c]
Cadmium	200	$>1.3\times10^6$(?)	<75(?)	2
Aflatoxin B$_1$	0.1	Epi: 10^4	5	8[c]
Ochratoxin A	1–3	7×10^4	5–20	2,4
Zearalenone	10^3	$2-5\times10^7$	10–25	2
Ethyl carbamate basal intake	20	10^7	1	7
+ wine drinking	100	10^7	5	7
+ spirit drinking	2×10^3	10^7	100	7
Benzene	100(?)	Epi: 7×10^6	0.7	6[c]
Tetrachloroethylene (PER)	<250(?)	10^8	<1	5[c]
Trichloroethylene (TRI)	50	10^9	0.021	5
1,1,1-Trichlorethane	85	5×10^8	0.085	5
Vinyl chloride	3	10^8	0.015	2
Styrene	10	5×10^8	0.01	2
Dimetridazole	<3(?)	10^8	0.015	9
Formaldehyde	2×10^4	$>>10^7$(?)	<<1,000(?)	1

[a]From experimental data (Gold *et al.*, 1984; 1986; 1987). Epi, from epidemiological data: arsenic and benzene (Becher and Wahrendorf, 1990); aflatoxin B$_1$ (Peers and Linsell, 1977).
[b]Reference from human intake in Switzerland. 1: Aeschbacher *et al.*, 1991; 2: Stähelin *et al*, 1991; 3: Shephard, 1991; 4: DFG, 1990; 5: Zimmerli *et al.*, 1982; 6: Lutz *et al*, 1991; 7: Schlatter and Lutz, 1990; 8: Dichter, 1984; 9: Voogd, 1981; 10: Kramers and Van Der Heijden, 1988.
[c]Assessment includes authors' evaluation.

One possibility to explain the discrepancy is the idea that important mutagenic dietary carcinogens have not yet been included in Table 1. Indeed, a large number of compounds of natural origin are not yet listed. Ames *et al.* (1990) estimated an average daily intake of 1.5 g natural "pesticides" per person. At this level on the order of mg/kg per day only low carcinogenic potencies (TD$_{50}$ of about 10^9 ng/kg per day) are required to produce appreciable calculated numbers of induced cancer cases (on the order of 1,000 per 1 million). We have not so far found published TD$_{50}$ estimates for these compounds but would welcome all contributions to complete Table 1.

Another possibility is an underestimation of the carcinogenic potencies derived from animal experiments. It could be argued that humans are more sensitive than rodents towards one or the other carcinogen.

A third possibility and, in our view, the most likely explanation of the above mentioned discrepancy, is the concept that *non*-mutagenic dietary constituents and endogenous processes are more important than dietary mutagens. This idea will be outlined below.

Non-mutagenic Dietary Carcinogens

A large number of dietary constituents increase tumour incidence in animal experiments without being mutagenic in short-term tests. These compounds have been shown to affect the stage of tumour promotion, most clearly after initiation of carcinogenesis by a genotoxic compound.

Such non-mutagenic carcinogens are compiled in Table 2, again with average human exposure levels and carcinogenic potency, if available. The cancer risk was estimated on the basis of the same assumptions made for the mutagenic carcinogens. It must be noted that a linear dose-response extrapolation is most likely too conservative for most of these carcinogens (Lutz, 1990b).

Most Important Risk Factor: Overnutrition

Epidemiological studies have shown an association between caloric intake, especially in the form of fat, and the occurrence of cancer at several sites, for instance in the breast, large bowel, and prostate.

In animals, it has been known for more than 50 years that dietary restriction results in a dramatic reduction of spontaneous and chemically-induced cancer incidence (review by Tannenbaum and Silverstone, 1953). Experiments published in 1942 (Tannenbaum, 1942) form the basis of the following attempt to attribute a "carcinogenic potency" to carbohydrate: One group of 50 female DBA mice was fed with 2 g of a mixture of dog chow meal and skimmed milk powder per mouse per day. Not a single breast tumour developed within 20 months. Another group received, in addition, cornstarch *ad libitum*. Average daily food consumption was 2.9 to 3.1 g, i.e. they consumed one gram of cornstarch in addition to the 2 g basic feed. In this group, the spontaneous breast cancer incidence within 20 months was 38 percent.

These data can be interpreted as if the additional gram carbohydrate per mouse per day was carcinogenic for the breast. Expressed in terms of a TD_{50}, the "carcinogenic potency" of cornstarch for the mouse mammary

Table 2 Non-mutagenic dietary carcinogens – risk estimation based on daily intake and daily dose resulting in 50% tumour incidence (TD_{50})

Compound	Human intake [ng/kg bw/d]	TD_{50}[a] [ng/kg bw/d]	Risk [cases per 10^6]	Ref[b]
Overnutrition	4×10^9 (as carbohydrate)	6×10^{10}	30,000	11
Ethanol	4×10^8	Epi: 5×10^{10}	$\leq4,000$	12
Sodium chloride	2×10^8	???	???	11
Saccharin	5×10^5	6×10^{10}	4	13
DEHP	2×10^3	2×10^9	0.5	14
Dieldrin	15	10^6–10^7	0.75–7.5	2
DDT isomers	30	10^7–10^8	0.15–1.5	2
$\alpha + \beta$ HCH	30	10^7	1.5	2
Captan	20	10^{10}	0.001	2
2,3,7,8 $TCDD_{eq}$	0.002	10^2–10^3	1–10	2

[a]From experimental data. Epi, from epidemiological data: ethanol (Doll and Peto, 1981).
[b]Reference for human intake in Switzerland. 2: Stähelin *et al.*, 1991; 11: Aebi *et al.*, 1984; 12: SFA, 1991; 13: Anonymous, 1991; 14: Bronsch, 1987.

gland, therefore, is about 60 g/kg per day, i.e. just as potent as sodium saccharin for the rat bladder (TD_{50}: 60 g/kg per day).

Average caloric intake (excluding alcohol) in Switzerland in 1985–87 was about 45 kcal/kg per day (Stähelin *et al.*, 1991). Basal requirements with light work are at 30 kcal/kg per day. Caloric overfeeding by 15 kcal/kg per day can be achieved with an excess of 4 g carbohydrate/kg per day. Taking into account a carcinogenic potency of TD_{50} = 60 g/kg per day, about 30,000 cancer cases in one million deaths could be attributed to caloric overnutrition (Table 2).

Obviously, overnutrition is not only due to carbohydrates but also to fat. Restriction of fat intake provided a similar protection from spontaneous tumour formation (Tannenbaum and Silverstone, 1953). Compared with carbohydrate, the "carcinogenic potency" of fat was somewhat higher, probably due to an additional tumour-promoting activity of fat not related to calories alone.

Caloric overnutrition appears to affect the late stages of carcinogenesis. Both experimental and epidemiological evidence support this view. (i) In the early experiments on the effect of dietary restriction on skin tumour induction by benzo[a]pyrene, caloric restriction had a much more pronounced effect on the promotion phase than on the initiation phase (Tannenbaum, 1944). (ii) Breast cancer mortality in England and Wales dropped by about 10 percent around 1940, almost simultaneously with a reduction in the consumption of meat and sugar (Ingram, 1981). Such an instantaneous effect is compatible with the idea that tumour progression was retarded, for instance by a reduced rate of cell division in the clones of transformed cells. This interpretation is important in the view of dietary recommendations. It means that stopping overnutrition has a beneficial effect at all ages and tumour stages.

High Risk Factors

The second ranking dietary carcinogen is ethanol. Epidemiologists attribute 2–4 percent of all cancer deaths in the USA to alcohol. Because of a multiplicative synergism with smoking, a maximum value of 1 percent is often attributed to alcohol alone (2,500 cases per 1 million, at an average yearly *per capita* consumption of 7 litre ethanol). Since the alcohol consumption in Switzerland is higher than in the USA, alcohol could account for up to 4,000 cancer cases per 1 million deaths.

Sodium, such as in the table salt sodium chloride, has tumour-promoting activity in animals for the bladder and the stomach. The worldwide decrease in stomach tumour incidence in humans in the last decades could at least in part be due to a reduction of the use of salt for conserving foods. We were not in a position to attribute a "carcinogenic potency" to sodium ions but would like to emphasize that even a low potency (e.g. a TD_{50} of about 10 g/kg bw, i.e. 10^{10} ng/kg per day) would suffice to generate a substantial risk because of the large amounts ingested.

Low Risk Factors

For the environmental contaminant 2,3,7,8-tetrachlorodibenzo [p] dioxin (TCDD) a risk of 1–10 in 1 million can be calculated. It is difficult to interpret this figure: on the one hand, a non-linear dose-response relationship would result in a lower risk, on the other hand, the longer half life of TCDD in humans as compared with rodents would result in higher tissue levels at comparable exposure levels.

Saccharin also ranks as a low risk factor in Table 2. We think that the actual risk is even smaller because we expect a sublinear dose-response.

Negligible Risk Factors

What has been said above for the mutagenic residues and contaminants also holds for the non-mutagenic ones. Residues of pesticides like DDT, dieldrin, hexachlorocyclohexane isomers (α- and β-HCH), captan, substances that migrate from packaging materials (plasticizers like bis(2,2'-

diethylhexyl)phthalate, DEHP), all represent negligible risks. If a non-linear dose–response relationship is assumed, the risk would be even lower.

Summary for Non-mutagenic Dietary Carcinogens

Table 2 shows that the risk from non-mutagenic dietary "carcinogens" could be very large if macronutrients are included in the evaluation. Caloric intake alone could be responsible for a large part of the cancer risk attributed to the diet. Alcohol and possibly salt are the next highest-ranking dietary non-mutagenic carcinogens. More data have to be collected to substantiate the assumption for sodium chloride.

It is interesting to note that the most important dietary carcinogens are of low potency (TD_{50} of grams per kg per day) but are ingested in large amount. Adaptive response of the organism to handle the gram amounts of compounds entails biological responses which probably alter the process of spontaneous carcinogenesis (Lutz, 1990a). On the other hand, for all substances where the human intake is low (milligrams and less) an adaptive response is not required so that no effect of the substance on spontaneous carcinogenesis is expected (unless the compound has hormonal activity).

Dietary Anti-carcinogens

A large body of epidemiological and experimental evidence illustrates the effect of nutritional deficiencies. The four main areas of interest are fibre, vitamins, minerals and inhibitors of carcinogenesis.

In the present context of quantifying different risk factors it is difficult to estimate a risk for the absence of a substance. This task is all the more complicated as high dose levels of anticarcinogens often turn out to be toxic (vitamin A) and/or carcinogenic (selenium, phenols). We cannot, therefore, include anti-carcinogens in our quantitative analysis but we mention this group in the view of recommendations to be made.

The concentration of anticarcinogens can be affected at all stages of food harvesting, storing, processing, and cooking. Disappearance of anti-carcinogens should, therefore, be avoided and supplementation could be discussed. For the latter, however, the evidence of a protective effect must have been shown over a wide dose range and should include spontaneous tumour formation.

Conclusions

Future Research Activities

Anything eaten in gram amounts is expected to have an effect on basic metabolic pathways and might require homeostatic adjustments in cells and tissues. An adaptive cellular response could entail changes in cell differentiation and thereby also affect the process of spontaneous carcinogenesis. We therefore recommend that all dietary high-level constituents should be more thoroughly investigated. In the class of the mutagenic carcinogens this includes a number of natural constituents as reviewed by Ames *et al.* (1990). In the class of the non-mutagenic carcinogens, table salt is a prime candidate.

Recommendations

Preamble: It should be noted that the same compound or group of compounds can originate from different sources (fat or salt as (i) a natural constituent, (ii) the result of industrial food processing, (iii) the result of cooking a meal). In such a situation, recommendations for the consumer should be backed up by regulations for farming, the food industry, and catering services.

1. DON'T OVEREAT. Substances that you eat in gram amounts are the most important risk factors to accelerate spontaneous carcinogenesis (fat, carbohydrates, protein). Restriction had a dramatic reducing effect on spontaneous tumour formation in animals.

2. EAT VEGETABLES, FRUITS, AND WHOLEMEAL PRODUCTS. An increase in the consumption of vegetables and fruits is recommended due to the presence of anti-carcinogens and fibre.

3. CUT DOWN ON ALCOHOL AND SALT. Alcohol and sodium chloride (table salt) rank second in terms of quantity. Reduction is highly recommended.

4. The formation of mutagenic carcinogens during food processing can be reduced by lowering cooking temperatures (microwave and steam instead of broiling). Simultaneously, decomposition of vitamins is reduced.

5. High doses of specific carcinogens in specific food items can be avoided by eating a varied, balanced diet.

6. Don't be afraid of traces of contaminants. They represent a negligible risk.

7.   ENJOY YOUR MEAL.

Note to reader: The authors do not consider the lists presented in this paper to be final. Readers are welcome to contribute new data, data which have been overlooked or which call for correction of our evaluation.

References

Anonymous (1991). Sweetener intakes. *Fd Chem Toxic* **29**: 71–72.
Aebi H, Blumenthal A, Bohren-Hoerni M, Brubacher G, Frey U, Müller HR, Ritzel G, Stransky M (Hrsg) (1984). Zweiter Schweizerischer Ernährungsbericht, Huber, Bern, Switzerland.
Aeschbacher HU (1991). Potential carcinogens in the diet. *Mutat Res* **259**: 203–410.
Ames BN, Profet M, Gold LS (1990). Dietary pesticides (99.99% all natural). *Proc Natl Acad Sci (USA)* **87**: 7777–7781.
Ames BN, Magaw R, Gold LS (1987). Ranking possible carcinogenic hazards. *Science* **236**: 271–280.
Becher H, Wahrendorf J (1990). Variability of unit risk estimates under different statistical models and between different epidemiological data sets. In: Scientific Issues in Quantitative Cancer Risk Assessment, SH Moolgavkar (ed), Birkhäuser, Basel, Switzerland, pp 267–285.
Bronsch C (1987). Untersuchungen zur Exposition und zum renalen Ausscheidungsverhalten des Kunststoffweichmachers Di(2-ethylhehyl)phtalat (DEHP) beim Menschen. Thesis No 8459, Swiss Federal Institute of Technology, Zürich, Switzerland.
DFG Deutsche Forschungsgemeinschaft (1990). Ochratoxin A Vorkommen und toxikologische Bewertung. VCH Verlagsgesellschaft mbH, Weinheim, Germany.
Dichter CR (1984). Risk estimates of liver cancer due to aflatoxin exposure from peanuts and peanut products. *Fd Chem Toxicol* **22**: 431–437.
Doll R, Peto R (1981). The causes of cancer: quantitative estimates of avoidable risks of cancer in the United States today. *J Natl Cancer Inst* **66**: 1191–1308.
Gold LS, Sawyer CB, Magaw R, Backman GM, de Veciana M, Levinson R, Hooper NK, Havender WR, Bernstein L, Peto R, Pike MC, Ames BN (1984). A carcinogenic potency database of the standardized results of animals bioassays. *Environ Health Perspect* **58**: 9–319.
Gold LS, de Veciana M, Backman GM, Magaw R, Lopipero P, Smith M, Blumenthal M, Levinson R, Bernstein L, Ames BN (1986). Chronological supplement to the carcinogenic potency database: standardized results of animal bioassays published through December 1982. *Environ Health Perspect* **67**: 161–200.
Gold LS, Slone TH, Backman G, Magaw R, Costa MD, Lopipero P, Blumenthal M, Ames BN (1987). Second chronological supplement to the carcinogenic potency database: standardized results of animal bioassays published through December 1984 and by the National Toxicology Program through May 1986. *Environ Health Perspect* **74**: 237–329.

Ingram DM (1981). Trends in diet and breast cancer mortality in England and Wales 1928–1977. *Nutr Cancer* **3:** 75–80.

Kramers PGN, Van Der Heijden CA (1988). Polycyclic aromatic hydrocarbons (PAH): carcinogenicity data and risk extrapolations. *Toxicol Environ Chem* **16:** 341–351.

Lutz WK (1990a). Endogenous genotoxic agents and processes as a basis of spontaneous carcinogenesis. *Mutat Res* **238:** 287–295.

Lutz WK (1990b). Dose-response relationship and low dose extrapolation in chemical carcinogenesis. *Carcinogenesis* **11:** 1243-1247.

Lutz W, Poetzsch J, Schlatter J, Schlatter Ch (1991). The real role of risk assessment in cancer risk management. *Trends Pharmacol Sci* **12:** 214–217.

Peers FG, Linsell CA (1977). Dietary aflatoxins and human primary liver cancer. *Ann Nutr Alim* **31:** 1005–1018.

Perera F, Boffetta P (1988). Perspectives on comparing risks of environmental carcinogens. *J Natl Cancer Inst* **80:** 1282–1291.

Schlatter J, Lutz WK (1990). The carcinogenic potential of ethyl carbamate (urethane): risk assessment at human dietary exposure levels. *Fd Chem Toxic* **28:** 205–211.

SFA (1991). Zahlen und Fakten zu Alkohol- und Drogenproblemen 1990/91. Schweizerische Fachstelle für Alkoholprobleme, Lausanne, Switzerland. ISBN 2–88183–027–7.

Shephard SE (1991). Risikobeurteilung von N-Nitrosoverbindungen un deren Vorläufer in der Nahrung. *Mitt Gebiete Lebensm Hyg* **82:** 36–44.

Stähelin HB, Lüthy J, Casabianca A, Monnier N, Müller HR, Schutz Y, Sieber R (Hrsg) (1991). Dritter Schweizerischer Ernährungsbericht. Bundesamt für Gesundheitswesen, Bern, Switzerland.

Tannenbaum A (1944). The dependence of the genesis of induced skin tumors in the caloric intake during different stages of carcinogenesis. *Cancer Res* **4:** 673–677.

Tannenbaum A, Silverstone H (1953). Nutrition in relation to cancer. *Adv Cancer Res* **1:** 451–501.

Voogd CE (1981). On the mutagenicity of nitroimidazoles. *Mutat Res* **86:** 243–277.

Zimmerli B, Zimmermann H, Müller F (1982). Perchlorethylen in Lebensmitteln. *Mitt Gebiete Lebensm Hyg* **73:** 71–81.

CHAPTER 3

Anticarcinogens/Inhibitors in the Diet

MJ HILL

ECP(UK)
38 East Street, Andover, Hants SP10 1ES, UK

Introduction

It was natural that most of the early interest in carcinogenesis should have centred on the identification of the *causes* of cancer and the *mechanisms* by which they act. It is also self-evident that the study of inhibitors of carcinogenesis had to await the identification of some causes and the establishment, in the light of such information, of model systems for cancer induction at specific sites and by specific mechanisms. Nevertheless, despite early work (e.g. Crabtree, 1947) and subsequent interest from key workers in the field of cancer research (e.g. Ames, 1983) the subject of anticarcinogenesis, the inhibition of carcinogenesis etc is not deemed worthy of separate listing in such listing journals as Index Medicus. Compare the lack of any journal of anticarcinogen research with the myriad of journals on carcinogenesis.

Crabtree (1947) defined an anticarcinogen as including "any factor, intrinsic or extrinsic, which delays or prevents the emergence of malignant characters in any tissue of any species of organism". This symposium is concerned with the human; consequently although most of the information in the literature is derived from animal work, only those substances for which there is evidence of activity in humans will be discussed here. The subject will be further constrained by the fact that the dietary anticarcinogens most widely explored, the vitamins and micronutrients, are discussed elsewhere in this symposium.

There are four principal routes by which anticarcinogens prevent carcinogenesis, these are:

(a) Scavenging and inactivating proximate carcinogens, precarcinogens or precursors of carcinogen formation.

(b) Preventing the proximate carcinogen or tumour promoter from reaching its target by, for example, blocking specific binding sites.

25

(c)   Preventing the action of proximate carcinogens by increasing the host cellular defences to mutation or transformation.

(d)   Preventing the development of precancerous lesions.

Anticarcinogens in food include macronutrients as well as micro-nutrients. The macronutrients include dietary fibre and vegetables; the latter may act principally via their vitamins and antioxidant micronutrients. The micronutrients include the polyols (e.g. tannins, gallic acid), synthetic antioxidants etc. In addition, there is a range of anticarcinogens produced in the colon by bacterial action on benign substrates; the most notable of these are the lignans, indoles and phenols.

In this review I will first discuss the "principal routes of action" identified above, and then will discuss some dietary sources of anticarcinogen in the context of these mechanisms.

Mechanisms of Anticarcinogenesis

In order that a compound can accomplish a chemical derivatization (particularly of the type implicated in chemical carcinogenesis) at room temperature it is necessary first to generate a high energy intermediate able to overcome the energy barrier to reaction. Such high energy inter-mediates are, by their nature, short-lived and are unlikely to have a high level of target specificity. Such reactants can interact with a range of compounds referred to collectively as antioxidants and, in this way, car-cinogenesis can be prevented before the carcinogen reaches its target. Target specificity is achieved before activation to the high energy state by facilitating entry of the carcinogen to the cell through the action of specific receptors. In consequence the carcinogen can be prevented from reaching the target by blocking or inactivating the specific receptor molecules. Cells are equipped with a wide range of detoxification mechanism and these are included in the array of mechanisms by which the cell expresses resistance to the action of toxic and genotoxic compounds. A further mechanism by which anticarcinogenic effects may be expressed is by the inhibition or reversal of precancerous lesions. In the stomach, for example, intestinal-type cancer is the culmination of a series of well-defined histological steps which begin with atrophic gastritis and then progress to intestinal meta-plasia and then through increasingly severe dysplasia to carcinoma. Anti-carcinogens could act to protect the gastric mucosa from the final stages by blocking any of the earlier stages.

Each of these mechanisms has been studied in depth, usually using the vitamins as the anticarcinogens (e.g. ascorbic acid or β-carotene as a free radical scavenger; ascorbic acid in protection against intestinal metaplasia of the stomach). They will now be discussed in turn using other food anticarcinogens as the examples.

(a) Scavenging and Inactivating Carcinogens and Precarcinogens

Most proximate carcinogens are highly active molecules, such as free radicals, potent electrophilic ions etc and can be scavenged and inactivated by a range of natural and synthetic antioxidants. The chemistry of this inactivation has been described by Wattenberg (1979, 1985) and more recently by Diplock (1988) and by Simic (1988). Examples of naturally occurring antioxidants are benzyl isothiocyanate, phenethylisothiocyanate and benzyl thiocyanate (all present in cruciferous vegetables; Virtanen, 1962); synthetic antioxidants include the food additives butylated hydroxyanisole (BHA) and butylated hydroxytoluene (BHT). The antioxidants of most interest have been the vitamins ascorbic acid and α-tocopherol and the provitamin β-carotene. A number of polyols present in the diet (e.g. gallic acid) are potent scavengers of nitrite – a precursor of the *N*-nitroso compounds.

(b) Inhibition of Transport Mechanisms

For a carcinogen to gain entry to the cell it needs to utilize some mechanism such as specific receptors, specific transport mechanisms etc. For example there are specific steroid hormone receptors in the breast, endometrium, and prostate and these are thought to be important in these hormone-dependent cancers (and also perhaps, in the colon where oestrogen binding sites have also been found). There is a family of phyto-oestrogens (Adlercreutz *et al*, 1987) which are able to block oestrogen-binding sites. In addition they may stimulate the production of steroid hormone binding globulin (SBHG), thereby again decreasing access of the steroid to the cell (Adlercreutz *et al.*, 1987). Inhibition of entry to the cell can be modulated by affecting the exposure levels by, for example, interfering with enterohepatic circulation (e.g. of oestrogens, thereby decreasing plasma levels) or by stool bulking (thereby decreasing the level of exposure of colon mucosal cells to luminal factors).

(c) Increase of Host Defence Mechanisms

Cells have a range of defence mechanisms; these include the mixed function oxidase (MFO) activity which is maximal in the liver but appears to be present in all tissues. These can be induced by a host of chemicals,

many of which are toxic themselves but many (such as flavones) which
have low toxicity (Wattenberg, 1979). β-naphthoflavone has been used to
increase MFO activity in the mouse lung and skin and the rat breast,
resulting in a decrease of the number of cancers induced by polycyclic
hydrocarbons. Cruciferous vegetables are rich in compounds able to
induce MFO activity, including a number of indoles (Loub *et al.*, 1975).

Some other naturally occurring compounds can cause decreased microsomal enzyme activity, including coumarin and a range of plant lactones,
and it has been postulated that this results in decreased activation of
carcinogen to proximate carcinogen and explains the inhibition of mammary cancer in a model system, or in the mouse forestomach (Wattenberg,
1979, 1985). Thus anticarcinogenic effects can be achieved by inhibiting
some enzymes and by stimulating others.

(d) Effect on Precancerous Lesions

In general the human host is remarkably resistant to carcinogens, but the
tissues in specific sites can be made more sensitive by the development of
precancerous lesions. Thus Barretts oesophagus greatly increases the risk
of adenocarcinoma of the oesophagus, intestinal metaplasia of the stomach greatly increases the risk of intestinal type gastric cancer, chronic
ulcerative colitis of more than 10 years duration greatly increases the risk
of colorectal cancer. Dietary factors which reverse these precursor lesions
can therefore be thought of as anticarcinogenic, albeit indirectly. The
causation and reversal of precursor changes have not been extensively
studied to date.

Anticarcinogenic Action of Dietary Components

A number of food items and macronutrients (e.g. vegetables, dietary fibre)
have been found from epidemiological studies to inhibit carcinogenesis.
Discussion of some of these in greater depth provides a useful method to
study anticarcinogenesis in greater depth.

Dietary Fibre

Numerous epidemiological studies have suggested a role for dietary fibre
in protection against cancer of the large intestine and of the breast.
Numerous hypotheses have been proposed to explain this observation,
but none has been subjected to rigorous study.

Butyrate production. The carbohydrate component of dietary fibre may be fermented by the gut bacterial flora, ultimately to short chain fatty acids, alcohol and gases. The short chain fatty acids result in a decreased colonic pH which results in the inhibition of a number of gut bacterial enzymes, including the 7-dehydroxylase that produces the secondary bile acids lithocholic and deoxycholic acids from the primary bile acids produced in the liver. The acid pH also decreases the solubility of the secondary bile acids. These two combine to cause a decreased concentration of the tumour promoting secondary bile acids in the colon and cause an amelioration of their dysplastic effect on the colon mucosa (Rafter *et al.*, 1986).

There is a body of evidence, based entirely on tissue culture studies, suggesting that butyrate has an anti-neoplastic effect; nobody to date has attempted to verify this in animal models by, for example, rectal instillation as used by Narisawa *et al.* (1974) to demonstrate tumour promotion by bile acids. However, it has been claimed that butyrate promotes colonocyte welfare and this, together with its anti-neoplastic effect, explains the protective effect of fibre. The only human study to date showed no difference in colonic butyrate concentration between colorectal cancer, colorectal adenoma and control patients. On *a priori* grounds a major difference between control and *adenoma* patients would be expected if the hypothesis had any validity (since inhibition of initiation is being proposed).

Source of phytate. Inositol hexaphosphate (phytic acid) is a common component of plant cell walls and, in many older methods of preparation, was a major contaminant of fibre and apparently responsible for many of its properties (e.g. cation binding, free radical scavenging etc).

Babbs (1990) has recently reviewed the evidence in favour of a role for free radicals in colon carcinogenesis, particularly hydroxyl radicals produced *in situ* in the colonic lumen by the superoxide-driven Fenton reaction. The major sources of the superoxide needed for this reaction are the gut bacteria; as usual most of the work has been done on the superoxide production by *Escherichia coli* (e.g. Hassan *et al.*, 1979) because, although the species usually represents less than 0.1% of the gut organisms, it is easy to grow. However it is certain that the dominant organisms also produce superoxide, and have the enzyme superoxide dismutase. The Fenton reaction requires the presence of ferric ions and, although most of the iron in the highly anaerobic colon is ferrous, it can be autoxidized to the ferric state by a host of gut bacterial pathways. Since phytate is a potent scavenger of ferric and ferrous ions it inhibits hydroxyl radical formation by the Fenton reaction; phytate also scavenges free radicals and so, by both of these pathways, should inhibit colon carcinogenesis initiated or promoted by hydroxyl radicals. This led Graf and Eaton (1985) to question whether the inhibition of experimental colon carcinogenesis was due to the carbohydrate "dietary fibre" component of the food or to the phytate content of fibre-rich foods. Shamsuddin *et al.* (1988) have reported suppression of experimental colon carcinogenesis in rats fed phytic acid; the model tumours were initiated by azoxymethane (AOM) in F344 rats. Phytate also decreased the mitotic activity in the crypts of the rat colonic mucosa; this is thought to be an early marker of subsequent colonic carcinogenesis. The phytate was protective whether the feeding was started before or 2 weeks after AOM initiation, and caused a decrease in colonic hydroxyl radical concentration.

Decrease carcinogen concentration. The distribution of colorectal cancers suggests that it is caused in part by a luminal factor that is concentrated (as a result of water recovery from the colon) during colonic transit. There have been many studies relating the risk of colorectal cancer to the concentration of putative carcinogens or promoters in the human colon (e.g. bile acids, ammonia, free radicals, nitrite etc). If this hypothesis is true then factors which dilute the colonic contents should protect against colorectal carcinogenesis. In accordance with this, the dietary fibre sources which offer the best protection against colon cancer in the animal models are those that provide the best stool bulking (particularly wheat bran and ispaghula). The importance of stool bulking has been discussed elsewhere (Hill and Fernandez, 1990); if this role is accepted then all stool-bulking foods should be considered as anticarcinogenic.

Many breast cancers, especially post-menopausal tumours are hormone-dependent, with the rate of their growth being dependent on circulating oestrogen concentrations in animal models. In accord with this, ablation therapy to remove the oestrogen sources (and so decrease the circulating oestrogen levels to nearly zero) has a recognized place in the surgical treatment of post-menopausal breast cancer. Oestrogens undergo enterohepatic circulation, with the vascular pool size being dependent in part on the rate of faecal loss. It has been demonstrated (Goldin *et al.*, 1982) that dietary fibre interferes with enterohepatic circulation of oestrogens by increasing their faecal loss and thereby decreasing their plasma concentration. It has been proposed that this is one of the methods by which a diet rich in dietary fibre decreases the risk of breast cancer; the evidence and arguments for this have been reviewed recently by Adlercreutz (1984; 1990).

Lignan production. The lignans are a family of compounds present in higher plants and which, in the last decade, have been increasingly often reported in the faeces of higher animals and humans (e.g. Stitch *et al.*, 1980; Adlercreutz *et al.*, 1981). They are diphenolic substances and are related to the plant isoflavonic phytoestrogens; they have been reviewed in detail elsewhere (e.g. Price and Fenwick, 1985). To date a total of 15 lignans and related compounds have been isolated from human urine but no doubt many more will be identified in the future; only a small number have been identified in significant quantities. Having identified such a group of phyto-oestrogen-related compounds the problem is now to identify their role. They are weak antioestrogens and bind to oestrogen receptors. It is therefore possible that they have an anticarcinogenic role in inhibiting oestrogen-dependent breast (and endometrial?) carcinogenesis. This hypothesis has been discussed in detail by Adlercreutz (1984; 1990) and could explain the protective role of dietary fibre against breast carcinogenesis. The role of lignans as potential anticarcinogens is complex; they are antiproliferative in tissue culture cell lines, and inhibit mutagen-induced proliferation of human lymphocytes (Hirano *et al.*, 1989), suggesting a possible role on cell proliferation and cell transformation.

Vegetables

In many early studies the role of vegetables in preventing human cancer was equated with that of dietary fibre. However more recent and sophisticated epidemiological studies have begun to dissociate the two and suggest a role for vegetables independent of its fibre content.

Fresh salad vegetables are rich in antioxidant vitamins and provitamins (retinoids, ascorbic acid, tocopherols, carotenes) and it is possible that these are responsible for the protective effect. As with dietary fibre the "protection" by the individual vitamins in epidemiological studies is less than that for vegetables, but that may be due to the inaccuracies involved in attempting to calculate vitamin intakes using food tables. A further possibility must be considered, and this is that the protection is not due only to the fibre, or only to the antioxidant vitamins etc, or even to a combination of all of these, but to some other anticarcinogenic component of vegetables.

For clues to the identity of such compounds it is necessary to return to the work of Wattenberg *et al.* already referenced earlier in this review.

Coumarins and lactones. These include the coumarins and umbelliferones that are common components of vegetables and fruits and which have been shown to inhibit experimental breast and gastric cancer (reviewed by Wattenberg, 1979).

Phenolic compounds. Plants contain a wide range of naturally occurring phenolic compounds, including the hydroxy-cinnamic acids, 3,4 dihydroxycinnamic acid (caffeic acid) which inhibit experimental gastric carcinogenesis and other experimental tumours produced by a wide range of carcinogens. Their mode of action is thought to be similar to that of the synthetic antioxidants BHA and BHT. Phenolic compounds are known to be active scavengers of such active anions as nitrite and to have potent antioxidant properties. However they also induce microsomal detoxification systems and so increase the cellular defences against genotoxic and cellular toxic agents.

Sulphur compounds. The cruciferous plants are a rich source of isothiocyanates; these have been shown to be active anticarcinogens in animal models of breast, lung and gastric cancer (Wattenberg, 1979). The mechanism of this inhibition is not known.

Indoles. Cruciferous vegetables are a rich source of a range of indoles (e.g. indole-3-carbinol, indole-3-acetonitrile) and these too, are potent anticarcinogens in models of cancer of the stomach and breast cancer. These compounds are known to stimulate microsomal mixed function oxidase activity against polycyclic aromatic hydrocarbons.

Implications for Dietary Advice

The loss of interest in anticarcinogenesis probably reflects a change in fashion rather than a considered judgment of the literature and it is probably much too soon to write off the importance of the concept of anticarcinogenesis. Nevertheless it needs to be recognized that such laboratory studies have their main value in rationalizing and supporting the results of epidemiology rather than in identifying *de novo* new foods that should be promoted in a healthy-eating campaign.

Before the ECP meeting in Aarhus there was a great deal of interest in cruciferous vegetables; this appears to have been transferred to salad vegetables, with better support from epidemiology.

If the results of epidemiology suggest that persons are protected if they eat more green vegetables or more foods rich in dietary fibre, and if these observations are not supported by the data on antioxidant vitamin consumption, then the explanation could be sought in the anticarcinogens considered here. However, in the opinion of this reviewer of the background literature, the evidence in favour of inhibition of carcinogenesis by antioxidant vitamins is very much stronger, and arguments in favour of dietary recommendations are much more likely to be found there.

References

Adlercreutz H (1984). Does fiber-rich food containing animal lignan precursors protect against both colon and breast cancer? An extension of the fiber hypothesis. *Gastroenterology* **86**: 761-6.

Adlercreutz H (1990). Western diet and western diseases: some hormonal and biochemical mechanisms and associations. *Scand J Lab Invest* **50**: (Suppl 201) 3–23.

Adlercreutz H, Fotsis T, Heikkinen R *et al.* (1981). Diet and urinary excretion of lignans in female subjects. *Med Biol* **59:** 259–61.

Adlercreutz H, Hockerstedt K, Bannwart C and 4 others (1987). Effect of dietary components, including lignans and phytoestrogens on enterohepatic circulation and liver metabolism of estrogens and on sex hormone binding globulin (SHBG). *J Ster Biochem* **27:** 1135–44.

Ames BC (1983). Dietary carcinogens and anticarcinogens. *Science* **221:** 1256–64.

Babbs CF (1990). Free radicals and the etiology of colon cancer. *Free Rad Biol Med* **8:** 191–200.

Crabtree HG (1947). Anticarcinogenesis. *Br Med Bull* **4:** 345–7.

Diplock AT (1988). Micronutrients and trace elements in cancer prevention. In *Gastric Carcinogenesis* (eds PI Reed, MJ Hill) Elsevier, Amsterdam, pp 99–104.

Graf E, Eaton JW (1985). Dietary suppression of colonic cancer – fiber or phytate? *Cancer* **56:** 717–8.

Hassan HM, Fridovich I (1979). Paraquat and Escherichia coli: mechanism of production of extracellular superoxide radical. *J Biol Chem* **254:** 10846-10852.

Hill MJ, Fernandez F (1990). Bacterial metabolism, fiber and colorectal cancer. In *Dietary Fiber* (eds D Kritchevsky, C Bonfield, J Anderson), Plenum, New York, pp 417–430.

Hirano T, Oka K, Akiba M (1989). Effects of synthetic and naturally-occurring flavonoids on mitogen-induced proliferation of human peripheral blood lymphocytes. *Life Sci* **45:** 1407–41.

Loub WD, Wattenberg LW, Davis DW (1975). Arylhydrocarbon hydroxylase induction in rats by naturally occurring inoles of cruciferous vegetables. *JNCI* **54:** 985.

Narisawa T, Magadia N, Weisburger J, Wynder EL (1974). Promoting effect of bile acids on colon carcinogenesis after intrarectal instillation of MNNG in rats. *JNCI* **53:** 1093–7.

Price KR, Fenwick GR (1985). Naturally occurring oestrogens in food. A review. *Fd Add Contam* **2:** 73–106.

Rafter JJ, Eng VWS, Furrer R, Medline A, Bruce WR (1986). Effects of calcium and pH on the mucosal damage produced by deoxycholic acid in the rat colon. *Gut* **27:** 1320–9.

Shamsudden AM, Elsayed AM, Ullah A (1988). Suppression of large intestinal cancer in F344 rats by inositol hexaphosphate. *Carcinogenesis* **9:** 577–580.

Simic MG (1988). Mechanisms of inhibition of free radical processes in mutagenesis and carcinogenesis. *Mutat Res* **202:** 377–86.

Stitch SR, Toumba JK, Groen MB *et al.* (1980). Excretion, isolation and structure of a phenolic constituent of female urine. *Nature* **287:** 738–40.

Virtanen AI (1962). Some organic sulfur compounds in vegetables and fodder plants and their significance in human nutrition. *Angew Chem Int Ed Engl* **1:** 299.

Wattenberg LW (1979). Naturally occurring inhibitors of chemical carcinogenesis. In *Naturally occurring carcinogens-mutagens and modulators of carcinogenesis* (eds EC Miller *et al.*). *Jap Soc Sci Press*, Tokyo, pp 315–29.

Wattenberg LW (1985). Inhibitors of carcinogenesis and their implications for cancer prevention in humans. In *Diet and Human Carcinogenesis* (eds Joossens J, Hill M, Geboers J); Excerpta Medica, Amsterdam, pp 49–60.

CHAPTER 4

Role of Vitamins and Micronutrients

EB THORLING

Danish Cancer Society
Department of Nutrition and Cancer, Norrebrogade 44,
DK-8000 Aarhus C, Denmark

Role of Vitamins and Micronutrients

We know of 13 vitamins, some appearing in different disguises (Friedrich, 1988) and a comparable number of important trace minerals (Prasad, 1976). Comprehensive review articles on these have been written by Dorgan and Schatzkin (1991) and by Creasey (1985).

I shall attempt, however, to give an overview of the subject, to draw a few conclusions and to cast some doubts on more established concepts and misconceptions.

A good place to start, if you want to investigate what kind of diet is ideal/appropriate for any kind of living being would be to look at its digestive apparatus.

A glance at the chewing machinery (and the digestive tract) of man immediately shows that man is not, and never was, a true carnivore. These teeth are not the grasping, cutting, chopping equipment of a wolf or a cat. On the other hand, nor is it the grinding millstones of a grass eater. The jaws appear well suited for roots and fruits, pulses and nuts but could well process smaller insects, worms, larvae, fish and clams. Only frying and cooking made meat masticable for man and it is not a coincidence that the chopped meat of hamburgers became a popular way of having the beef.

Another good way to gain information on the ideal diet is to scrutinize the biochemical potential of the body to look for possible deficiencies in synthetic capability. Apparently we have lost some synthetic pathways during the evolution. The most conspicuous in this connection is the loss of L-gluconolactone oxidase which is necessary for the synthesis of ascorbic acid. This defect is shared with the anthropoid apes, the guinea pig and the bats. Fish, however, also lack the ability to synthesize ascorbic acid. We must consequently rely on the synthetic capabilities of other living organisms to compensate for these lost pathways (e.g. bacteria and moulds are responsible for most of the synthesis of vitamin B12). We call the end products of these lost pathways the vitamins.

From a chemical point of view all vitamins are very different and they represent many classes of chemicals. When it comes to cancer they could not be expected to react in a uniform way nor to be of equal importance. In fact just a few so far seem to be of any importance for the development of cancer in man.

Where the minerals are concerned they must all be supplied from exogenous sources, some in large quantities (e.g. sodium, potassium, magnesium and calcium), some in smaller amounts (e.g. iodine and iron) and some in micro amounts to meet the needs of the organism. For cobalt a few milligrams mean the difference between life and death. Just as was the case for vitamins, the minerals enter into a multitude of different mechanisms in the normal function of the cells and the relation to cancer is apparent for just a few of these minerals. It is, however, a strange selection of rather few minerals that nature has chosen for life and it is likely that still more minerals will be shown in the future to be of vital importance even in minute amounts.

Some minerals are toxic, some extremely so and some are believed to be carcinogenic such as nickel, cadmium and hexavalent chromium (IARC, 1980). In a number of cases the evidence for carcinogenicity is, however, still questionable. In fact we should not assign carcinogenic properties to any specific element. Nickel is no more carcinogenic than is carbon. However, certain nickel compounds and many carbon compounds are extremely so.

A pertinent question when it comes to essential micronutrients is of course: what is the required daily average dose? (Benito, 1992). The answer that you get will, of course, depend on how you ask, required for what? The generally accepted RDA's (recommended daily allowances) is the dose that will prevent any deficiency symptoms to appear in most normal healthy adults (Gaby, 1991) (separate values for children). Even here we still see some discrepancies between countries as for instance in the recommended dose of vitamin C which varies from 50 to 200 mg per day. This dose, however, may not be sufficient for everyone, smokers require 4 times the RDA to acquire an acceptable blood concentration, and of course the dose does not cover disease states. The RDA value is, however, believed to be well below the general toxic level.

Some of the vitamins and most of the essential minerals are indeed toxic in higher doses (Evans and Lacey, 1986). Usually it is not so difficult to determine this toxic level and to stay clear of it. From a nutritional point of view, however, the most interesting dose is not the minimal required dose or the toxic dose but what has been termed with the elusive name the "optimal dose", believed to be somewhere in between these two extremes.

Now here the really interesting discussion begins with the definition of "optimal", again starting with the question: optimal for what?

We are inclined to believe that the ideal diet is the diet that will give us perfect health (whatever this may be – when absence of disease is secured) and to allow for a strong fast-growing generation of young people. In this respect we have learned a lot from the veterinarians who are indeed very good at producing a lot of flesh in the shortest possible time and at the cheapest price! The veterinarians, however, know only very little of old age since most of their clients will never attain this goal so attractive for most humans. Now – is it really so that a healthy adolescence and a strong large body will also assure a long life and less cancer (and other chronic diseases) in old age? No – "it ain't necessarily so".

Animal experiments and epidemiological evidence support the general experience from carcinogenesis studies that larger animals (of a particular species) and increased height in man poses an increased risk of cancer (Albanes and Taylor, 1990). Better nutrition throughout adolescence means more cell divisions, more mitoses (since cell size is not increased) and increased proliferative activity is known to increase the risk of cancer (Ames and Gold, 1990b; Cohen and Ellwein, 1990). Better nutrition, vitamins and minerals have led to an increase in body size in most western countries and in Japan over the last few decennia of up to 20 cm in height and about an equal number of kilos. It is not fair to ascribe this to any isolated effect of a particular vitamin and/or mineral, fat or protein but to a combined effect of some complexity. At the same time we see the girls mature at an earlier age with menarche occurring in still younger girls. One consequence is a longer interval between menarche and the birth of the first child – childbirth being postponed for a number of "cultural" reasons. This would mean an increased risk of mammary cancer, a trend readily observed.

It is known that proliferative activity in any one organ or specific cell type increases the probability for cancer development in this particular tissue (Cohen and Ellwein, 1990; Ames and Gold, 1990a). The most likely explanation is that possible errors in the DNA are "fixed" during the mitosis and that the probability of mutations is thereby increased. Another explanation could be that – if Hayflick's theory is accepted – proliferation means "aging" (Goldstein, 1990). The more stem cells that are triggered into proliferation, the older the tissue. This means that the normal organism may very well have "an asynchronous cell/organ aging", making the chronological age of the individual less important than the biological age of his organs. If for instance the liver is constantly triggered into proliferation by say alcohol, aflatoxin or hepatitis, this liver would age fairly rapidly compared to non-affected livers. You may consequently have a young person with an old liver – and an increased risk of liver cancer.

Some vitamin deficiencies are known to be accompanied by a decreased cell survival and an increased reparative cell replacement. This would mean an increased risk of cancer.

For the survival of the human race it is, of course, important to have healthy young people to breed healthy children. There is, however, little evolutionary selective benefit in having a large generation of older people without cancer. There is apparently no selective pressure to promote a cancer-free senescence. Cancer incidence rates only start to increase in a logarithmic way after the end of the reproductive years. In most wild-living populations it might easily be seen as an advantage for the species to get rid of members above the reproductive age, competing for the same food and territory as the breeding generations. We like to believe that all of us slightly older members of society may still be of some value for our human race. Nature may not agree – and cancer may be one way to make us step down from the stage.

Getting back to the vitamins and the micronutrients an exciting picture is beginning to shine through (Diplock, 1991). Only a limited number of these compounds appears to be protective against the development of cancer in experimental systems and from epidemiological studies. Most of these appear to be involved in the antioxidative defences against oxygen-derived radicals (Diplock, 1990; Miller, 1989; Special Communication, 1991).

Depending upon our physical activity, man reduces about 20 moles of oxygen to water per day or about 600–700 grams. This takes place at a temperature of 37 degrees Celsius and at a partial pressure of from 100 to 40 mm mercury. This indeed is a very risky business. Oxygen is an extremely reactive element. The invention about 3 billion years ago of the oxidative metabolism, with all its energy dependent advantages, necessitated a concomitant development of a multitude of defence mechanisms to make this possible. Most of the oxygen in the animal organism is reduced in the mitochondrial electron transport pathways which secure the least possible release of free radicals with unpaired electrons. In spite of this a fairly sizable fraction of the oxygen will generate intermediate oxygen radicals. These compounds especially the hydroxyl radical are extremely reactive and have attracted an increasing attention in recent years. Our understanding of their deleterious effect is increasing.

To protect us from most of the toxic effects, the cells contain a number of defence systems of varying effectiveness and importance, working in concert as backup mechanisms for each other. In the aqueous phase the most important compound is vitamin C, ascorbic acid, and the sulfhydryl groups of the aminoacids in proteins and polypeptides such as glutathione. In the lipid phase of the cell membranes we have especially vitamin E, the tocopherols. Furthermore, cells contain a number of enzyme systems that participate at different levels, such as the superoxide dismutases, the peroxidases and catalase. It is of interest here that these enzymes are dependent for their function on exactly those minerals that were found to be protective in animal experiments, etc. Most conspicuous may be selenium as part of glutathione peroxidase.

These antioxidants and protective enzyme systems may consequently protect us against most of the effects from oxygen-derived radicals. However, the protection is not 100 per cent. Ames and colleagues have estimated that in spite of these systems our cells will still suffer damage to their DNA, a damage that amounts to 10,000 base oxidations per cell per day in man and many more in smaller animals such as mice and rats with larger oxygen turnover (Ames and Saul, 1985; Cathcart *et al.*, 1984). Rancidification of lipids in our cell membranes is minimized by the presence of vitamin E and repair is made by the selenium-containing glutathione peroxidase. Deficiencies in vitamin E and selenium are characterized by an increased rancidification of cell membrane lipids with a distortion of the membrane organisation and receptor systems and consequently signal perception (Van Vleet and Ferrans, 1989).

The toxicity of the oxygen-derived radicals is on the other hand utilized by our organism in the killing of germs by the leucocytes (Baehner *et al.*, 1982). White blood cells produce a burst of radicals when they have ingested bacteria and the germs are then killed by the damage to their cell surface proteins and lipids.

Plants had to invent the carotenes to protect themselves against the oxygen-derived radicals produced in the photosynthesis (Di Mascio *et al.*, 1991). It is interesting that these carotenes may also be protective in the animal organism. Best known is the beta-carotene, best because it is the most abundant and because the analytical procedures are relatively simple and easy compared to some of the other carotenes. Some of these (there are scores of them) may nevertheless be equally important in plants as well as in animals.

Now – it is to be expected that nature "has tried to" optimize the performance of the antioxidative defence systems. It requires energy and resources to synthesize the enzymes involved and it takes energy to quench the effect of the radicals. Cells cannot afford to set aside for these activities more than what turns out to be absolutely necessary since a multitude of other tasks have to be performed to assure the integrity and well functioning of the cell. Now: What is enough?

From a biological point of view enough is just sufficient to assure that the individual lives long enough to reproduce itself and create a healthy offspring. It is interesting that in the reproductive organs testis and ovary, the antioxidative systems are particularly active.

The consequence is that some damage is accepted as inevitable – inescapable – could cancer be one of these consequences?

There are two questions to be answered when it comes to the possible advantage that we make of this new knowledge even at this fairly early stage with so much still being hypothetical. The first is concerned with the possibly increased risk of cancer in persons who are deficient, overt, borderline or subclinical in one or more of these factors.

We have two lines of evidence for this of which the case/referent studies are the most frequent and the least reliable and the cohort studies which are theoretically better but rare and expensive. The final "proof" would be the prospective intervention studies of which a number are currently under way (Holm, 1990; Meyskens and Prasad, 1986). It appears from these lines of evidence that borderline deficiency in vitamin C, E provitamin A, selenium and zinc should be avoided since in all probability a resulting low activity of the antioxidant status is likely to increase our risk of cancer. I say this mindful of all the pitfalls in interpreting the basic reports from the epidemiologist and the animal researchers. Especially when it comes to the ingestion of plant food it is obvious that by eating plants we ingest thousands of active chemicals some known, most of them still unknown that might interfere with action of the few that have been described so far in more details (Ames, 1983). This takes me right to the second question, the possible beneficial effect of larger "pharmacologic" doses of the "protective" factors. We have no solid human experience to justify this so far. On the other hand, it is conceivable that certain risk groups would benefit from, e.g. the protective effect of beta-carotene, vitamins C and E and maybe selenium, but this remains to be supported in further studies. Again we should remember that the oxygen-derived radicals play an important role in the way we stay clear of bacterial infections and that there is a limit to how far we can go in our attempts to eliminate them completely.

Remember rabbits get cancer – and they even produce their own ascorbic acid – and so do plants. I will end on a more poetic note with the proposal for contemporary guidelines for good dietary habit:

FRUITS AND ROOTS

A DISH OF FISH

GREEN AND ROUGH

IS FINE ENOUGH

NIBBLE CHEESE

REFRAIN FROM GREASE

TAKE A LITTLE MEAGRE MEAT

WINE, A CUP TO MAKE IT NEAT

THIS, INDEED, IS ALL YOU NEED

References

Albanes D, Taylor PR (1990). International differences in body height and weight and their relationship to cancer incidence. *Nutrition and Cancer* **14:** 69–77.

Ames BN (1983). Dietary carcinogens and anticarcinogens. Oxygen radicals and degenerative diseases. *Science* **221:** 1256–1264.

Ames BN, Gold LS (1990a). Dietary carcinogens, environmental pollution, and cancer: some misconceptions. *Med Oncol and Tumor Pharmacother* **7:** 69–85.

Ames BN, Gold LS (1990b). Too many rodent carcinogens: mitogenesis increases mutagenesis. *Science* **249:** 970–971.

Ames BN, Saul RL (1985). Oxidative DNA damage, aging and cancer. In *Diet and Human Carcinogenesis*. Proceedings of the 3rd Annual Symposium of the European Organization for Cooperation in Cancer Prevention Studies (ECP), Aarhus, Denmark, June 19–21, 1985. (eds Joossens JV, Hill MJ, Geboers J); Excerpta Medica, Amsterdam, New York, Oxford, pp 25–34.

Baehner RL, Boxer LA, Ingraham LM (1982). Reduced oxygen by-products and white blood cells. In *Free Radicals in Biology*, Volume V (ed Pryor WA); Academic Press, Orlando, pp 91–113.

Benito E (1992). Overview of dietary recommendations. *Public Education on Diet and Cancer* (eds. Benito, E, Giacosa, A. and Hill, MJ), Kluwer Academic Publishers, Lancaster. p. 3–12.

Cathcart R, Schwiers E, Saul RL, Ames BN (1984). Thymine glycol and thymidine glycol in human and rat urine: A possible assay for oxidative DNA damage. *Proc Natl Acad Sci USA* **81:** 5633–5637.

Cohen SM, Ellwein LB (1990). Cell proliferation in carcinogenesis. *Science* **249:** 1007–1011.

Creasey WA (1985). Diet and Cancer. Lea & Febiger, Philadelphia, pp109–159.

Di Mascio P, Murphy ME, Sies H (1991). Antioxidant defence systems: the role of carotenoids, tocopherols, and thiols. *Am J Clin Nutr* **53:** 194S-200S.

Diplock AT (1990). Mineral insufficiency and cancer. *Med Oncol and Tumor Pharmacother* **7:** 193–198.

Diplock AT (1991). Antioxidant nutrients and disease prevention: an overview. *Am J Clin Nutr* **53:** 189S-193S.

Dorgan JF, Schatzkin A (1991). Antioxidant micronutrients in cancer prevention. Hematology/Oncology Clinics of North America. *Nutrition and Cancer* **5:** 43–68.

Evans CDH, Lacey JH (1986). Toxicity of vitamins: complications of a health movement. *Br Med J* **292:** 509–510.

Friedrich W (1988). Vitamins. Walter de Gruyter, Berlin, New York.

Gaby SK, Bendich A, Singh VN, Machlin LJ (Eds) (1991): Vitamin Intake and Health. A Scientific Review. Marcel Dekker, Inc., New York.

Goldstein S (1990). Replicative senescence: The human fibroblast comes of age. *Science* **249:** 1129–1132.

Holm L-E (1990). Nutritional intervention studies in cancer prevention. *Med Oncol and Tumor Pharmacother* **7:** 209–215.

IARC (1980). IARC Monographs on the Evaluation of the Carcinogenic Risk of Chemicals to Humans, Vol. 23, Some Metals and Metallic Compounds, Lyon.

Meyskens FL Jr, Prasad KN (1986) (Eds): Vitamins and Cancer. Human Cancer Prevention by Vitamins and Micronutrients. Humana Press, Clifton, New Jersey.

Miller AB (1989). Vitamins, minerals and other dietary factors. In *Diet and the Aetiology of Cancer* (ed Miller AB); Monographs, European School of Oncology. Series Editor: U. Veronesi. Springer-Verlag, Berlin, Heidelberg, pp 39–54.

Prasad AS (1976) (Ed): Trace Elements in Human Health and Disease. Volume 1 and 2. Academic Press, New York.

Special Communication (1991). Vitamin C: Biologic functions and relation to cancer. *Nutrition and Cancer* **15**: 249–280.

Van Vleet JF, Ferrans VJ (1989). Myocardial and pancreatic damage in selenium-vitamin E deficient mice. In *Selenium in Biology and Medicine* (ed Wendel A); Springer-Verlag, Berlin, Heidelberg, pp 142–150.

CHAPTER 5

Animal Studies on Diet and Cancer: are They of Value?

AP MASKENS

ECP, Avenue Lambeau 62, 1200 Brussels, Belgium

Introduction

Animal data are frequently referenced when attempts are made to establish dietary recommendations for humans. This paper will discuss the value and limits of such comparisons or extrapolations.

The aim therefore will not be to review animal data in specific fields of diet and carcinogenesis since such aspects will, in fact, be covered by other speakers. Rather, we will make use of one specific example, colon cancer in rodents, to analyse the nature of information produced by animal experiments, and conclude on their potential implications for human situations. We will also draw some conclusions in terms of public education.

Diet Experiments in Rodent Colon Carcinogenesis

The Nature of Carcinogenesis

Carcinogenesis is a biological phenomenon expressed by the emergence of one or several cancers, and the end-result of diet experiments will be the number of cancers eventually produced using different dietary regimens in conjunction with bowel-specific chemical carcinogens. Each such cancer is the consequence of one completed set of specific genetic changes having occurred in one single cell of the colorectal mucosa.

Kinetic analyses of chemical carcinogenesis in the colon of rodents have indicated that probably two consecutive specific changes must occur in the genome of single epithelial cells to allow for the expression of malignant properties, one resulting from the mutagenic effect of the chemical inducer, and the other allowing for the expression of the first, recessive, change. This second step can result from either an additional mutation, or a mitotic error converting the recessive mutant to a homozygous state. It

43

is worth noting that each of these two steps remain rare events. For instance, in BD IX rats given weekly injections of 1,2 dimethylhydrazine (DMH) at a dose of 9 mg per kg (or 2.7×10^{19} alkylating molecules), the incidence of cancers will be as low as 1.4×10^{-8} per cell at risk per dose of DMH per year. This figure is extremely stable and reproducible within given experimental settings (Maskens, 1981).

The object of dietary experiments will precisely be to obtain changes in this incidence rate by modifying the diet of animals submitted to standard carcinogen treatments.

The Nature of Dietary Changes

Dietary changes are by nature very different from the process of carcinogenesis. While carcinogenesis is a process initiated at the level of DNA in single cells, diet relates to behavioural and physiological functions at the level of the entire organism. Dietary changes will therefore involve varied and multiple direct and indirect physiological consequences, of which those affecting the carcinogenesis risk may well be difficult to identify.

Thus, common experiments in which changes are forced at the level of fat or fibre contents of rat diets will have as consequences:

–   general changes (e.g. total calories intake, hormonal metabolism)

–   digestive physiology changes (e.g. bile secretion)

–   intestinal physiology changes (e.g. faecal bulk and contents, microflora)

–   mucosal changes (cell renewal rate).

Each of these can in turn combine with others to produce additional modifications. Thus, alterations in the microflora can interact with the bile compounds to produce co-carcinogenic metabolites, which in turn will interact differently with the mucosal cells of the colon according to their proliferative status (Thompson and Hill, 1987).

What can we Conclude from Animal Experiments?

Of course, some of the diversity observed in dietary experiments reported in the literature, has largely to do with the absence of common and comparable experimental protocols (animal strain) (Wilpart, 1987). An example is given in Table 1, reviewing experimental data on fibre and colorectal carcinogenesis (from Hill, 1985). But then the complex nature of diet and its consequences will add to the difficulty in interpreting the observed data. And even when conclusions seem to be fairly consistent

Table 1 Rat model

Type of fibre	Carcin-ogen	Route	Sex of rats	Effect	Reference
Cellulose (29% or 40%)	AOM	Sc	M	None	Watanabe *et al.*,1979
Cellulose	DMH	Sc	M	Protect	Trudel *et al.*, 1983
Cellulose 15%	DMH	Oral	M	None	Kritchevsky 1986
Hemicellulose	DMH	Sc	M	None	Freeman *et al.*, 1984
Hemicellulose	DMH	Oral	M	Protect	Kritchevsky, 1986
Bran (20%)	DMH	Oral	M	Protect	Kritchevsky, 1986
Bran (20%)	DMH	Sc	M	None	Kritchevsky, 1986
Bran	DMH	Sc		Promote	Jacobs, 1984
Bran (20%)	DMH	Oral	F	None	Kritchevsky, 1986
Carrot (20%)	DMH	Sc	M	Promote	Kritchevsky, 1986
Pectin (15%)	MNU	IR	F	None	Watanabe *et al.*, 1979
Pectin (15%)	AOM	Sc	F	Protect	Watanabe *et al.*, 1979
Pectin	DMH	Sc	M	Promote	Bauer *et al.*, 1979

DMH: 1,2-dimethylhydrazine
AOM: azoxymethane
MNU: methylnitrosourea

and coherent, can we derive conclusions applicable to humans? In other words, when we conclude from rat observations that a 15% pectin-rich diet can be predictably associated with a decrease in tumour production in azoxymethane-treated female F344 rats (Watanabe *et al.*, 1979), does it mean we should propose this diet to humans? Asking the question is giving the answer.

However, such experiments can provide answers to more fundamental questions which are in fact relevant to humans. They do for instance tell us that under certain conditions, dietary changes can and do modify cancer risk. Also, inasmuch as animal experiments can be conducted to a very deep level of analysis, they can be used to demonstrate which biochemical or physiopathological mechanisms are at the basis of the modulation of cancer risk, thus providing useful indications for directions in which to explore the human situation.

To continue the example of the colon cancer experiments, animal studies have shown that a variety of factors which enhance cell proliferation in the colorectal epithelium do in fact potentiate the carcinogenic effect of chemical carcinogens. Such factors include, for instance, bile acids

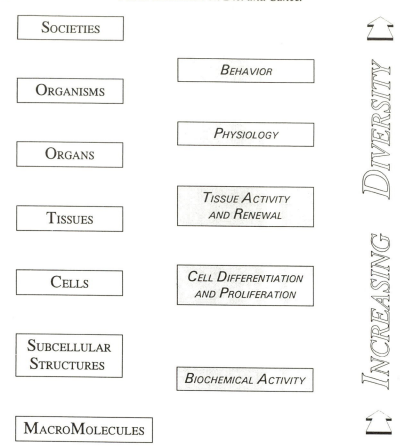

Figure 1

(Reddy *et al.*, 1976; Deschner and Raicht, 1979; Reddy and Watanabe, 1979; Cohen *et al.* 1980), non-specific injury (Pozharisski, 1975), or transmissible murine colonic hyperplasia (Barthold and Jonas, 1977). As some of the dietary changes implicated in promotion of the experimental cancers can also, via indirect routes, increase the proliferative activity of the epithelium (Jacobs, 1984), we can derive possible mechanisms. This information can now be exploited in the human situation, where increased proliferative activity has also been observed to be associated with increased cancer risk (Deschner and Maskens, 1982; Maskens, 1987). What can however be transposed to the human situation is not the potential action of the specific diet given to the experimental animals, but rather the human transposition of the same fundamental mechanisms. Thus, these observations could lead to attempting to verify, in humans, (1) whether some human diets do in fact increase the proliferative activity in the colon, and (2) whether such diets will in fact be associated with increased cancer risk.

Thus, while animal experiments can be useful in pointing at basic mechanisms potentially applicable in the human situation, their specific conclusions can by no means be directly translated at the level of human diet. At this second level, animal experiments need to be complemented by human data, coming from case control studies including clinical as well as dietary investigations, and, better, from prospective intervention studies.

The main point here is that, while colon cells or crypts from rats are very similar to those of humans, this resemblance decreases as we increase the complexity level at which we operate. The organisms are indeed very different, and so are the behaviours (Figure 1). Thus, while similarities can exist at the most basic levels (e.g. cell proliferation) of the mechanisms demonstrated in the animals, it is not at all certain that the higher level phenomena (e.g. diet) capable of initiating these mechanisms will be comparable.

Two additional reasons for not translating the conclusions of animal studies directly to man, are that:

1.   The chemical carcinogenesis induction of the tumours in rats represents *per se* a highly specific situation, not reproduced *per se* in the natural human environment. One injection of DMH certainly represents a highly toxic event, with a high proportion of cell destruction in the colorectal mucosa, important liver damage, and other toxic effects.

2.   The human diet is varied and difficult to control, as opposed to the strict regimens used in experiments.

Conclusions

In answer then to the question in the title of this presentation, we will thus conclude that:

1.   Animal studies have been very useful in confirming that dietary changes can modify cancer risk. They are similarly of great interest in demonstrating some of the fundamental mechanisms by which dietary changes can induce such modifications.

2.   Animal studies are of no value in the definition of specific human dietary recommendations. They must therefore be complemented by human observations.

Consequences in terms of public education.   Since, however, human observations cannot reach the level of scientific certitude obtained in animal experiments, we will have to accept that we must base our dietary recommendations on the best available evidence, and, perhaps, never on full scientific proof.

The need for further human research.   Simultaneously, we will have to improve the value of human data by the organization of large scale studies, possibly prospective in nature. Europe, with its wide diversity of cultures and dietary habits, represents a remarkable opportunity for such projects, in which ECP will hopefully continue to play an active role.

References

Barthold SW, Jonas AM (1977). Morphogenesis of early 1,2-dimethylhydrazine-induced lesions and latent period reduction of colon carcinogenesis in mice by a variant of Citrobacter freundii. *Cancer Res* 37: 4352–4360.

Bauer HG, Asp N, Oste R, Dahlquist A, Redlund P (1979). Effect of dietary fiber on the induction of colorectal tumours and β-glucuronidase activity in the rat. *Cancer Res* 39: 3752–3756.

Cohen BI, Raicht RF, Deschner EE, Takahashi M, Sarwal AN, Fazzini E (1980). Effect of cholic acid feeding on N-methyl-N-nitrosourea-induced colon tumors and cell kinetics in rats. *J Natl Cancer Inst* 64: 573–578.

Deschner EE, Maskens A (1982). Significance of the labeling index and labeling distribution as kinetic parameters in colorectal mucosa of DMH-treated animals and cancer patients. *Cancer* 50: 1136–1141.

Deschner EE, Raicht RF (1979). Influence of bile on kinetic behaviour of colonic epithelial cells of the rat. *Digestion* 19: 322–327.

Freeman HJ, Spiller GA, Kim YS (1984). Effect of high hemicellulose corn-bran in 1,2-dimethylhydrazine-induced rat intestinal neoplasia. *Carcinogenesis* 5: 261–264.

Hill MJ (1989). Experimental studies of fat, fiber and calories. In *Diet and Etiology of Cancer* (ed Miller AB); Springer, Heidelberg, pp 31–38.

Jacobs LR (1984). Stimulation of rat colonic crypt cell proliferative activity by wheat bran consumption during the stage of 1,2-dimethylhydrazine administration. *Cancer Res* 44: 2458–2463.

Kritchevsky D (1986). Fiber and cancer. In *Dietary Fiber: Basic and Clinical Aspects* (eds Vahouny G, Kritchevsky D); Plenum, New York, pp 427–432.

Maskens A (1981). Confirmation of the two-step nature of chemical carcinogenesis in the rat colon adenocarcinoma model. *Cancer Res* 41: 1240–1245.

Maskens A (1987). The polyp/cancer sequence in the large intestine. In *Causation and Prevention of Colorectal Cancer* (eds Faivre J, Hill MJ) Excerpta Medica, Amsterdam, pp 39–48.

Pozharisski K (1975). The significance of nonspecific injury for colon carcinogenesis in rats. *Cancer Res* 35: 3824–3830.

Reddy BS, Narisawa T, Weisburger JH and Wynder EL (1976). Promoting effect of sodium deoxycholate on colon adenocarcinomas in germ-free rats. *J Natl Cancer Inst* **56:** 441–442.

Reddy BS and Watanabe K (1979). Effect of cholesterol metabolites and promoting effect of lithocholic acid in colon carcinogenesis in germ-free and conventional F344 rats. *Cancer Res* **39:** 1521-1524.

Trudel JL, Senterman MK and Brown RA (1983). The fat fiber antagonism in experimental colon carcinogenesis. *Surgery* **94:** 691-696.

Watanabe K, Reddy BS, Weisburger JH and Kritchevsky D (1979). Effect of dietary alfalfa, pectin, and wheat bran on azoxymethane- or methylnitrosourea-induced colon carcinogenesis in F344 rats. *J Natl Cancer Inst* **63:** 141–145.

Wilpart M (1987). Dietary fats and fiber and experimental colon carcinogenesis: a critical review of published evidences. In *Causation and Prevention of Colorectal Cancer* (eds Faivre J, Hill MJ); Excerpta Medica, Amsterdam, pp 85–98.

PART TWO
UPDATE PAPERS

CHAPTER 6

Diet and Colorectal Cancer

J FAIVRE

Registre des Tumeurs Digestives (Equipe associée INSERM-DGS)
Faculté de Médecine, 7 Boulevard Jeanne d'Arc
21033 Dijon Cédex, France

Colorectal cancers are responsible for a very high morbidity and mortality throughout the world, being one of the commonest cancers in industrialized countries whereas other countries display very low incidence rates (Muir *et al.*, 1987). There is a lot of evidence for attributing most of the differences between countries to environmental factors, in particular to dietary factors. Migrant studies (Locke and King, 1980) and studies of religious sub-groups with special dietary habits (Jensen, 1983) have given considerable support to this hypothesis. The first studies which pointed out a particular food or nutrient in relation to colorectal carcinogenesis were correlation studies comparing dietary habits between high and low risk areas. But hypotheses needed to be confirmed in studies at the individual level, case-control, cohort and intervention studies.

Fat, Protein, Meat and Large Bowel Cancer

One of the strongest correlations between diet and colorectal cancer incidence was with total fat, total protein and per capita meat intake (Armstrong and Doll, 1976; Gregor *et al.*, 1969; MacKeon-Eyssen and Bright-See, 1984). Things are unfortunately less clear when analysing case-control studies. Out of 15 studies which considered the association between large bowel cancer and fat intake, ten found an increased risk for total fat or saturated fat intake (Bristol *et al.*, 1985; Freudenheim *et al.*, 1990; Graham *et al.*, 1988; Jain *et al.*, 1980; Kune *et al.*, 1987; Lyon *et al.*, 1987; Martinez *et al.*, 1981; Philips, 1975; Slattery *et al.*, 1988; West *et al.*, 1989), and five failed to find any such relationship (Benito *et al.*, 1991; Dales *et al.*, 1978; Macquart-Moulin *et al.*, 1986; Philips, 1985; Tuyns *et al.*, 1987). As for protein, seven studies found an increased risk with high protein intake (Benito *et al.*, 1991; Freudenheim *et al.*, 1990; Jain *et al.*,

1980; Lyon *et al*, 1987; Potter *et al*., 1982; Slattery *et al*., 1988; West *et al*., 1989) and five found no effect (Bristol *et al*., 1985; Graham *et al*., 1988; Kune *et al*., 1987; Macquart-Moulin *et al*., 1986; Tuyns *et al*., 1987). A high consumption of meat was reported as a risk factor in 9 case-control studies (Bjelke, 1974; Haenszel *et al*., 1973; Jain *et al*., 1980; Kune *et al*., 1987; La Vecchia *et al*., 1988; Manousos *et al*., 1983; Martinez *et al*., 1981; Philips, 1975; Young and Wolf, 1988) over 15. Only 8 studies considered the role of fish in the aetiology of large bowel cancer: four studies found a high consumption of fish to be protective (Bjelke, 1974; Haenszel *et al*., 1973; Kune *et al*., 1987; La Vecchia *et al*., 1988), whereas one study considered it to be a risk factor (Graham *et al*., 1978), and three studies found no effect (Dales *et al*., 1978; Macquart-Moulin *et al*., 1986; Tuyns *et al*., 1987). In a prospective US study (Willett *et al*., 1990), colon cancer was positively associated with beef, pork, lamb, processed meats and liver whereas fish and chicken without skin displayed an inverse relationship. The high fat diet hypothesis drew considerable support from the well designed and well analysed study performed in Toronto by Miller and Jain (Jain *et al*., 1980; Miller *et al*., 1983). Total fat, total protein and saturated fat displayed a dose effect relationship with the risk of colorectal cancer. In multivariate analysis, the strongest association was with saturated fat both in males and females. It is interesting to note that whereas most positive studies come from North America or Australia, little association between fat and large bowel cancer is observed in West European studies. This may be due to real differences on risk factors rather than the methodological problems.

In experimental studies, the incidence of chemically induced large bowel cancers increased with the amount of fat in the diet. The animals given a 20–30% fat diet had a higher incidence of colon tumours than those given a 5–15% fat diet (Bansal *et al*., 1978; Broitman *et al*., 1977; Bull *et al*., 1979; Nauss *et al*., 1983; Nigro *et al*., 1979; Reddy and Hirot, 1979; Reddy and Mori, 1981; Reddy *et al*., 1976). Several experimental protocols have studied the influence of the nature of the fat (Nauss *et al*., 1983; Nauss *et al*., 1984; Reddy and Hirot, 1979). At a 5% level a greater number of large bowel tumours were found in rats fed with polyunsaturated fat than in rats fed with saturated fat. At a 20–30% level the effect on tumorigenesis was the same whatever the type of fat. The few studies taking into account the stage of carcinogenesis during which the dietary fat content was modified suggest a promoting effect of fat (Broitman *et al*., 1977; Nigro *et al*, 1979; Reddy and Hirot, 1979; Wilpart and Roberfroid, 1987).

Fibre and Large Bowel Cancer

Burkitt, comparing the high incidence of large bowel cancer in western countries with the low incidence rates in Africa suggested that most of the difference could be due to the lack of dietary fibre in westernized diet (Burkitt, 1971). Unfortunately, little is known on per capita fibre consumption and only four recent correlation studies were able to take into account dietary fibre, i.e. carbohydrates that are not digested in the human gastro-intestinal tract (Bingham *et al.*, 1979; Jensen *et al.*, 1982; MacKeon-Eyssen and Bright-See, 1984; MacLennan *et al.*, 1978). The results of analytical studies are still rather contradictory. There are ten case-control studies supporting a protective effect of dietary fibre (Benito *et al.*, 1991; Bjelke, 1974; Dales *et al.*, 1978; Freudenheim *et al.*, 1990; Heilbrun *et al.*, 1989; Kune *et al.*, 1987; Lyon *et al.*, 1987; Modan *et al.*, 1975; Tuyns *et al.*, 1987; West *et al.*, 1989), seven studies which found no effect (Bristol *et al.*, 1985; Dales *et al.*, 1978; Graham *et al.*, 1988; Jain *et al.*, 1980; Lee *et al.*, 1989; Macquart-Moulin *et al.*, 1986; Pickle *et al.*, 1984) and two studies indicating an increased risk associated with a high fibre intake (Martinez *et al.*, 1981; Potter *et al.*, 1982). In a nested case-control study from a cohort of Japanese who emigrated in the US, a protective effect of dietary fibre was observed only in low fat intake men (Heilbrun *et al.*, 1989). In a prospective study in US women, fibre from fruit was found protective against colon cancer (Willett *et al.*, 1990).

Dietary fibre is not a homogeneous entity and different components may have different physiological effects. Some components may be more efficient than others as protective agents against cancer. The lack of data in food composition tables concerning the different types of dietary fibre may explain why the results of epidemiological studies are rather contradictory. The findings from a sophisticated correlation study in Denmark and Finland stressed that dietary fibre should not be considered as a whole (Jensen *et al.*, 1982). The consumption of pentosans was higher in the low risk population than in the high risk population. A similar trend was observed for the hexose fraction. This was not the case for the uronic acid fraction of the non starch polysaccharides and cellulose.

During the last decade many reports have been concerned with the influence of dietary fibre in chemically initiated experimental carcinogenesis mainly in rats. Some investigations have examined the effect of a single source of fibre. Out of 14 experimental protocols presented within eight papers (Bauer *et al.*, 1979; Bauer *et al*, 1981; Castleden, 1977; Freeman *et al.*, 1980; Jacobs and Lupton, 1986; Klurfeld, 1987; Reddy *et al.*, 1981; Watanabe *et al.*, 1979) on the effect of dietary pectin on large bowel tumorigenesis, 3 displayed evidence of tumour inhibition. In three other experiments, tumour enhancement was demonstrated, while eight other protocols showed no effect of pectin. Concerning cellulose, 9 papers were published concerning 19 experimental protocols (Freeman *et al.*, 1978; Jacobs and Lupton, 1986; Klurfeld, 1987; Nigro *et al.*, 1979; Prizont, 1987; Ward *et al.*, 1973; Wilpart, 1987). Two experiments suggested an increased risk with a high consumption of cellulose, 9 no effect and 8 a decreased risk. But when taking into account only the experiments in which cellulose was given during the promoting phase there was no reduction in tumour incidence. These data imply that cellulose may protect against tumorigenesis only at the initiating period. Mucilaginous substances, like Fybogel®, (isphaghula fibre) appear to have a protective effect (Wilpart, 1987). Interestingly the protective effect of Fybogel® on carcinogenesis was observed during the promoting phase. Guar-gum, (Bauer *et al.*, 1981; Castleden, 1977; Jacobs and Lupton, 1986; Klurfeld, 1987) alfalfa (Nigro *et al.*, 1979; Watanabe *et al.*, 1979), carrageenan (Watanabe *et al.*, 1979) or cutin (Klurfeld, 1987) seemed to have no effect on large bowel carcinogenesis or even to increase the risk.

Concerning bran the effect varies with the bran source. Corn bran (Barnes *et al.*, 1983; Freeman *et al.*, 1980; Reddy *et al.*, 1985), rice bran (Castleden, 1977), soybean bran (Barnes *et al.*, 1983), oat bran (Jacobs and Lupton, 1986) do not seem to be protective. Wheat bran seems more interesting (Abraham *et al.*, 1980; Barbolt and Abraham, 1978; Barbolt and Abraham, 1980; Barnes *et al.*, 1983; Bauer *et al.*, 1981; Cruse *et al.*, 1978; Fleiszer *et al.*, 1978; Jacobs, 1983; Nigro *et al.*, 1979; Reddy *et al.*, 1981; Reddy *et al.*, 1983; Watanabe *et al.*, 1979; Wilson *et al.*, 1977). A protective effect was found in all studies where the diet contained 2–6% fat. The results vary in rats given a high fat diet. Available data also suggest that wheat bran might be more effective during the promoting phase than during the initiating phase (Nauss *et al*, 1984).

So it is apparent from animal studies of dietary fibre and colon cancer that attention should be focused on differentiating the types of fibres. They can have an enhancing effect, a protective effect, or no effect on large bowel carcinogenesis depending on the nature, amount, form of the fibre, and on the period of administration. Mucilaginous substances and wheat bran appear to be of particular interest. But interpretation of the data is difficult because they have been provided by various experimental protocols in which dietary fibre was administered to rats belonging to various strains, treated by carcinogens differing in nature and amount, with differences in the composition of diet, sometimes not even corrected for isocaloricity. Furthermore different tumorigenic parameters have been used as end point. There is an urgent need for animal models studies to be standardized to the greatest feasible extent. Efforts are also made to provide the detailed composition in dietary fibre of the most important food items. This will enable the epidemiologists to reanalyse their data and provide a better understanding of the relationship between human colorectal carcinogenesis and dietary intake fibre. Finally, the relevance of all these data to primary prevention of colorectal cancer will have to be determined by intervention studies involving dietary fibre supplementation.

Vegetables, Fruits and Large Bowel Cancer

One of the most interesting and consistent findings of analytical studies is the protective effect of vegetables. In 13 (Benito *et al*, 1990; Bjelke, 1974; Graham *et al*., 1978; Haenszel *et al*., 1980; Jain *et al*., 1980; Kune *et al*., 1987; La Vecchia *et al*., 1988; Macquart-Moulin, 1986; Manousos *et al*., 1983; Philips, 1975; Tuyns *et al*., 1988; West *et al*., 1989; Young and Wolf, 1988) out of 16 case-control studies, and in two out of three cohort studies (Hirayama, 1985; Philips and Snowdon, 1983) patients with large bowel cancer had a lower consumption of vegetables than cancer-free controls. In a study in Marseille the protective effect of vegetables was limited to colon cancer, whereas no effect was observed for rectal cancer (Macquart-Moulin *et al*., 1986). In a study in Belgium there was a strong protective effect of vegetables against both colon and rectum cancer and it was stronger for raw vegetables than for cooked vegetables (Tuyns *et al*., 1987). In Western New York significantly reduced risks for colon cancers were observed for high consumption of tomatoes, peppers, carrots, onions and celery, but not for cruciferous vegetables (Graham *et al*., 1988), whereas other studies showed that the cancer cases had a particularly low intake of cruciferous vegetables. The study among Hawaiian Japanese was the only one to show a weak positive relationship between colon cancer and some vegetables: string beans and peas (Haenszel *et al*., 1973).

Only six case-control studies considered the role of fruit in the aetiology of colorectal cancer. Bjelke found a reduced risk for a high consumption of fruit both in Minnesota and in Norway (Bjelke, 1974), whereas no significant association was seen in the five other case-control studies (Kune *et al*., 1987; Macquart-Moulin *et al*., 1986; Manousos *et al*., 1983; Pickle *et al*., 1984; Tuyns *et al*., 1988).

Vitamins, Minerals and Large Bowel Cancer

Several vitamins and minerals have been suggested to be protective against large bowel cancers.

Vitamin A (retinol) and its provitamin β carotene have been shown experimentally to suppress the malignant transformation induced by chemical carcinogens on several cell lines. They could also prevent the chemical induction of animal tumours *in vivo*. The association of colorectal cancer risk with vitamin A intake was evaluated in six case-control studies (Bristol *et al*., 1985; Graham *et al*., 1988; Kune *et al*., 1987; La Vecchia *et al.*, 1988; Macquart-Moulin *et al.*, 1986; Potter *et al.*, 1982). No association with risk of colorectal cancer was found in five, one found an increased risk in relation to retinol but no association with β carotene (Tuyns *et al.*, 1988).

Some experimental and epidemiological studies have suggested a role for Vitamin C in the prevention of large bowel cancer. In Reddy's and Hirot's experiment, supplementation with sodium ascorbate inhibited DMH-induced large bowel carcinogenesis in rats (Reddy *et al.*, 1977). In case-control studies a negative association of vitamin C with colorectal cancer was found in six studies (Freudenheim *et al.*, 1990; Heilbrun *et al.*, 1989; Kune *et al*, 1987; Macquart-Moulin *et al.*, 1986; Potter *et al.*, 1982; West *et al.*, 1989), but no association was reported in six other studies (Bristol *et al.*, 1985; Graham *et al.*, 1978; Graham *et al.*, 1988; Jain *et al.*, 1980; La Vecchia *et al.*, 1988; Tuyns *et al.*, 1988). There is only limited clinical evidence suggesting the efficacy of ascorbic acid as a chemopreventive agent in patients with polyposis coli.

No information is available from epidemiological studies concerning vitamin E. A protective effect of this vitamin against chemically induced colon tumours has been suggested.

Some evidence for a protective effect of vitamin D and calcium has been recently drawn from epidemiological and experimental studies. In the United States a consistent inverse relationship between calcium intake and colon cancer mortality in the different states was observed both for men and women (Garland and Garland, 1980). Among seven case-control studies which studied the relationship between calcium intake and large bowel cancer, six showed no effect of calcium (Freudenheim *et al.*, 1990; Graham *et al.*, 1988; Kune *et al.*, 1987; Macquart-Moulin *et al.*, 1986; Negri *et al.*, 1990; Tuyns *et al.*, 1987) and one a protective effect of high calcium consumption (Slattery *et al.*, 1988). Support for the hypothesis was obtained from a 19-year prospective study in the USA (Garland *et al.*, 1985). In this study the risk of colorectal cancer was inversely correlated with dietary intake of vitamin D and calcium. This result was not confirmed in another cohort study in Hawaii (Stemmermann *et al.*, 1984), but the method of collecting dietary data was only a 24-hour recall which is too rough to study dietary intake at the individual level. In a case control study considering the patterns of milk consumption (Mettlin *et al.*, 1990), whole milk drinking was associated with an increased risk of colon and rectum cancers but low fat milk consumption had a protective effect on rectal cancer.

Enhanced epithelial proliferation in the bowel has been observed in patients at high risk for large bowel cancer. Oral calcium supplementation has been demonstrated to induce a more quiescent equilibrium of epithelial-cell proliferation in the colonic mucosa of subjects at high risk of colon cancer, similar to that observed in subjects at low risk (Lipkin and New-mark, 1985; Rozen *et al.*, 1989).

Alcohol and Large Bowel Cancer

An international study in which several environmental variables were correlated with cancer mortality and incidence led to the suggestion that beer consumption might be of aetiological importance in rectal cancer. The same correlation with beer also held for the different states in the US (Breslow and Enstrom, 1974). Trends for rectal cancer in the United Kingdom, Australia and New Zealand also correlated with beer consump-tion. In the IARC coordinated study in Finland and Denmark, alcohol consumption was positively associated with large bowel cancer incidence (MacLennan *et al.*, 1978).

Studies of alcoholics have shown conflicting results. In Denmark no increased risk was found among brewery workers, who on average drink four to five times as much beer as the general population (Jensen, 1979). By contrast a similar study of brewery workers in Ireland showed a doubling of the risk of rectal cancer (Dean *et al.*, 1979). Differences in beer composition that could result from brewing practices or from the compo-nents of the beer itself might explain these apparently conflicting results.

Among case-control studies beer was found to be a risk factor for rectal cancer in five studies (Freudenheim *et al.*, 1990; Kabat *et al*, 1986; Kune *et al.*, 1987; Miller *et al.*, 1983), although in one (Kabat *et al.*, 1986) the authors thought the relationship could be due to incomplete control for con-founders. In two other studies increased risk with beer consumption was limited to colon cancer. In another study (Potter and MacMichael, 1986) total alcohol intake (but not especially beer) was associated with an increased risk of both colon and rectal cancer. The relationship appeared to be stronger in males than in females. Six case-control studies have failed to show any association between alcohol and large bowel cancer (Benito *et al.*, 1990; Bjelke, 1974; Dales *et al*, 1978; Graham *et al.*, 1988; La Vecchia *et al.*, 1988; Manousos *et al*, 1983).

In two prospective cohort studies the risk of rectal cancer has been increased with total alcohol use. In one of them, the positive association with consumption of alcohol was limited to beer drinkers whose usual monthly consumption of beer was 15 litres or more (Pollack *et al.*, 1984). The other study suggested that total alcohol use, but no specific beverage type, was associated with increased risk of rectal cancer (Barbolt and Abraham, 1980). In a 17-year cohort study in Japan (Hirayama, 1989) a close association was observed between cancer of the sigmoid colon and alcohol consumption with a relative risk for drinkers vs non drinkers of 4.38 in men and 1.92 in women. The attributable risk in men was estimated as high as 74%. The highest risks were observed for daily beer drinkers but other drinks such as sake and shochu also displayed a strong relationship with the risk of sigmoid cancer.

In a cohort of Japanese men in Hawaii (Stemmermann *et al.*, 1990) rectal cancer was found to be strongly associated with alcohol intake both as total amount and as a percent of total calories and beer was the only alcoholic beverage that displayed a dose–response relationship. Colon cancer was also found to be associated with alcohol but only as a percent of caloric intake. The authors suggested that alcohol might displace cancer inhibitors from the diet.

Diet and Large Bowel Adenomas

There has been so far only two published studies on the role of diet in the occurrence of colorectal adenomas (Hoff *et al.*, 1986; Macquart-Moulin *et al.*, 1987). The first study was carried out on 77 cases and an equal number of controls enrolled in a screening programme concerning a population sample of 400 subjects of Norway aged 50–59 (Hoff *et al.*, 1986). The results indicated a higher intake of carbohydrates and fibre for controls and a higher intake of fat for cases. This study was well designed, but has the inconvenience of a rough statistical analysis comparing only mean values, without adjustment for confounders, in particular caloric intakes. The second study, performed in Marseille (France), was based on 250 cases and 250 controls (Macquart-Moulin *et al.*, 1987). The intake of polysaccharides and natural sugar was lower among cases than among controls, the risk of colorectal adenomas decreasing linearly with increasing daily consumption. In contrast sugar added to food and drinks was observed to have the opposite effect i.e. an increasing risk with increasing consumption. The cases also reported a lower consumption of oil, potatoes, K, Mg and vitamin B6. Unfortunately none of those studies took into account the multi-stage concept of the adenomas-carcinoma sequence. According to this hypothesis factors causing the development of adenoma *per se* should differ from those influencing the growth of the small adenoma into a larger one and from those inducing malignant change. This has important implications in that large bowel cancer could be modulated at different stages of its development. The inconclusive results of analytical epidemiological studies relating diet to large bowel cancer could be explained, at least partly by the fact that precancerous states have not been taken into account in most studies. This hypothesis is now investigated in two studies which are in progress (Faivre, 1986; Riboli, 1986).

The most consistent data on the relationship between colorectal tumours and diet come indirectly from biochemical studies focused on bile acids. Metabolic epidemiological and histopathological studies in humans, experimental studies in rodents and *in vitro* studies have provided data relating the faecal bile acid concentration to the risk of large bowel cancer. In some of those, a detailed analysis has been conducted considering the profile of individual faecal bile acids. The ratio of lithocholic to deoxycholic acids has been shown to be higher in cancer cases than in controls. Regarding that ratio significant differences could also be observed between the large adenoma group (>5 mm) and the small adenoma group (Owen *et al.*, 1987). Such data suggest that the secondary bile acids, lithocholic acid and deoxycholic acid, and mainly their ratio, are important in the step of growth phase of the adenoma i.e. in cancer promotion. They do not seem to play a role in the formation of small adenomas.

Some evidence was published recently in the role of alcohol and tobacco on the risk of large bowel adenomas. In England (Cope *et al.*, 1991), current smoking was more common in the adenoma group than in the control group and teetotallers were more common in the control group. Both drinking and current smoking led to a RR of 12.7 compared to total abstainers. In Japan (Kono *et al.*, 1990), the association between adenomatous polyps of the sigmoid and alcohol intake was limited to sake and beer with a dose-response relationship. In the US (Kikendall *et al.*, 1989) cumulative smoking and cumulative beer consumption were both associated with adenomas. Unfortunately again none of these studies considered the location nor the size of the adenoma. In a study of diet and colorectal tumours set up in Burgundy (unpublished data), there was an association between both alcohol and tobacco consumption and the risk of large adenomas whereas tobacco was the main difference between small adenomas and polyp-free controls. A multi-stage process involving tobacco for adenoma formation and alcohol for adenoma growth could be proposed. When considering polyp location, tobacco seemed to act at any site of the large bowel whereas alcohol seemed to be mainly involved in the growth of left colon adenomas.

Conclusion

Evidence from descriptive epidemiological studies and animal experiments have led to the suggestion that nutritional factors play an important role in the aetiology of large bowel cancer. Evidence from case control studies or prospective studies provide defensible arguments for dietary implications in the causation of large bowel cancer either as initiators and promoters or as inhibitors of carcinogenesis. There is fairly consistent evidence of the protective effect of vegetables. There is some evidence relating fat intake, fibre intake or calcium intake to cancer of the large bowel. Available data are not sufficient to serve as a basis for strong specific dietary advice and studies on large bowel cancer should be undertaken, particularly in the field of intervention studies.

References

Abraham R, Barbolt TA, Rodgers JB (1980). Inhibition by ban of the colonic cocarcinogenicity of bile salts in rat given dimethylhydrazine. *Exp Mol Pathol* **33:** 133–143.

Armstrong B, Doll R (1976). Environmental factors and cancer incidence in different countries, with special reference to dietary practices. *Int J Cancer* **15:** 617–631.

Bansal SR, Rhoads SE, Bansal SC (1978). Effects of diet on colon carcinogenesis and the immune system in rats treated with 1,2 dimethylhydrazine. *Cancer Res* **38:** 3923–3303.

Barbolt TA, Abraham R (1978). The effect of bran on dimethylhydrazine-induced colon carcinogenesis in the rat. *Proc Soc Exp Biol Med* **157:** 656–659.

Barbolt TA, Abraham R (1980). Dose response, sex difference and the effect of bran in dimethylhydrazine induced intestinal tumorigenesis in rats. *Toxicol Appl Pharmacol* **55:** 417–422.

Barnes DS, Clapp NK, Scott DA, Oberst DL, Berry SS (1983). Effect of wheat, rice, corn and soybean bran on 1,2-dimethylhydrazine induced large bowel tumorigenesis in F344 rats. *Nutr Cancer* **5:** 1–9.

Bauer HG, Asp NG, Oste R, Dahlqvist A, Fredlund PE (1979). Effect of dietary fiber on the induction of colorectal tumors and fecal β-glucuronidase activity in the rat. *Cancer Res* **39:** 3752-3756.

Bauer HG, Asp NG, Dahlqvist A, Fredlund PE, Nyman M, Oste R (1981). Effect of two kinds of pectin and guar gum on 1,2-dimethylhydrazine initiation of colon tumors and on fecal β-glucuronidase activity in the rat. *Cancer Res* **41:** 2518–2523.

Benito E, Obrador A, Stiggelbout A, Bosch FX, Mulet M, Munoz N, Kaldor J (1990). A population-based case-control study of colorectal cancer in Majorca. I. Dietary factors. *Int J Cancer* **45:** 69–76.

Benito E, Stiggelbout A, Bosch FX, Obrador A, Kaldor J, Mulet M, Munoz N (1991). Nutritional factors in colorectal cancer risk: a case-control study in Majorca. *Int J Cancer* **49:** in press.

Bingham S, William DR, Colet J, James WP (1979). Dietary and regional large bowel cancer mortality in Britain. *Br J Cancer* **40:** 456–63.

Bjelke E (1974). Epidemiological studies of cancer of the stomach, colon and rectum; with special emphasis on the role of diet. *Scand J Gastroenterol* **9: Suppl 31** 1–235.

Breslow NE, Enstrom JE (1974). Geographic correlations between cancer mortality rates and alcohol tobacco consumption in the United States. *JNCI* **53:** 631–639.

Bristol JB, Emmett PM, Heaton KW, Williamson RCN (1985). Sugar, fat, and the risk of colorectal cancer. *Br Med J* **291:** 1467–1470.

Broitman SA, Vitale J, Varrousek-Jakuba E, Gottlich LS (1977). Polyunsaturated fat: cholesterol and large bowel tumorigenesis. *Cancer* **40:** 2455–2463.

Bull AW, Soullier BK, Wilson PS, Hayden MT, Nigro ND (1979). Promotion of azoxymethane-induced intestinal cancer by high fat diet in rats. *Cancer Res* **39:** 4956–4959.

Burkitt DP (1971). Epidemiology of cancer of the colon and rectum. *Cancer* **28:** 3–13.

Castleden WM (1977). Prolonged survival and decrease in intestinal tumors in dimethylhydrazine-treated rats fed a chemically defined diet. *Br J Cancer* **35:** 491–495.

Cope GF, Wyatt JI, Pinder IF, Lee PN, Heatley RV, Kelleher J (1991). Alcohol consumption in patients with colorectal adenomatous polyps. *Gut* **32:** 70–72.

Cruse JP, Lewin MR, Clark CG (1978). Failure of bran to protect against experimental colon cancer in rats. *Lancet* **2:** 1278–1280.

Dales LG, Friedman GD, Ury HK, Grossman S, Williams SR (1978). A case control study of relationships of diet and other traits to colorectal cancer in American blacks. *Am J Epidemiol* **109:** 132-144.

Dean G, MacLennan R, McLoughlin H, Shelly E (1979). The causes of death of blue-collar workers at a Dublin brewery. *Br J Cancer* **40:** 581–589.

Faivre J (1986). In Muir CS, Wagner G eds. Directory of on going research in cancer epidemiology. IARC Scientific publications No 80. Lyon, IARC p103.

Fleiszer D, Murray D, MacFarlan J, Brown R (1978). Protective effect of dietary fibre against chemically-induced bowel tumours in rats. *Lancet* **2:** 552–553.

Freeman HJ, Spiller GA, Kim YS (1978). A double-blind study on the effect of purified cellulose dietary fiber on 1,2-dimethylhydrazine-induced rat colonic neoplasia. *Cancer Res* **38:** 2912–2917.

Freeman HJ, Spiller GA, Kim YS (1980). A double-blind study on the effect of differing purified cellulose and pectin fiber diets on 1,2-dimethylhydrazine-induced rat colonic neoplasia. *Cancer Res* **40:** 2661–2665.

Freeman HJ, Spiller GA, Kim YS (1984). Effect of high hemicellulose corn bran in 1,2-dimethylhydrazine-induced rat intestinal neoplasia. *Carcinogenesis* **5:** 261–264.

Freudenheim JL, Graham S, Marshall JR, Haughey BP, Wilkinson G (1990). A case-control study of diet and rectal cancer in western New York. *Am J Epidemiol* **131:** 612–624.

Freudenheim JL, Graham S, Marshall JR, Haughey BP, Wilkinson G (1990). Lifetime alcohol intake and risk of rectal cancer in western New York. *Nutr Cancer* **13:** 101–109.

Garland C, Garland F (1980). Do sunlight and vitamin D reduce the risk of colon cancer? *Int J Epidemiol* **9:** 227–231.

Garland C, Shekelle RB, Barrett-Connor E, Criqui MH, Rossof AM, Paul O (1985). Dietary vitamin D and calcium and risk of colorectal cancer: a 19-year prospective study in men. *Lancet* **7:** 307-309.

Graham S, Dayal H, Swanson M (1978). Diet in the epidemiology of cancer of the colon and rectum. *JNCI* **61:** 709–714.

Graham S, Marshall J, Haughey B, Mittelman A, Swanson M, Zielezny M, Byers T, Wilkinson G, West D (1988). Dietary epidemiology of cancer of the colon in western New-York. *Am J Epidemiol* **128:** 490–503.

Gregor O, Toman R, Frusona F (1969). Gastrointestinal cancer and nutrition. *Gut* **10:** 1031–1034.

Haenszel W, Berg JW, Kurihara M, Locke F (1973). Large bowel cancer in Hawaiian Japanese. *JNCI* **51:** 1765–1799.

Haenszel W, Locke FB, Segi M (1980). A case control study of large bowel cancer in Japan. *JNCI* **64:** 17–22.

Heilbrun LK, Nomura A, Hankin JH, Stemmermann GN (1989). Diet and colorectal cancer with special reference to fiber intake. *Int J Cancer* **44:** 1–6.

Hirayama T (1985). Diet and cancer: feasibility and importance of prospective cohort study. In: Joosens JV, Hill MJ, Geboers J eds. Diet and human carcinogenesis. Amsterdam, Elsevier pp191-198.

Hirayma T (1989). Association between alcohol consumption and cancer of the sigmoid colon: observations from a Japanese cohort study. *Lancet* **23:** 725–727.

Hill MJ, Morson BC, Bussey HJR (1978). Aetiology of adenoma-carcinoma sequence in the large bowel. *Lancet* **1:** 245–247.

Hoff G, Moen E, Trygg K, Frolich W, Sauar J, Vatn M, Gjones E, Larsen S (1986). Epidemiology of polyps in the rectum and sigmoid colon. Evaluation of nutritional factors. *Scand J Gastroenterol* **21:** 199–204.

Hoff G, Foerster A, Vatn MH, Sauar J, Larsen S (1986). Epidemiology of polyps in the rectum and colon. Recovery and evaluation of unresected polyps 2 years after detection. *Scand J Gastroenterol* **21:** 853–862.

Jacobs LR (1983). Enhancement of rat colon carcinogenesis by wheat bran consumption during the stage of 1,2-dimethylhydrazine administration. *Cancer Res* **43:** 4057–4061.

Jacobs LR, Lupton JR (1986). Relationship between colonic luminal pH, cell proliferation and colon carcinogenesis in 1,20-dimethylhydrazine treated rats fed high fiber diets. *Cancer Res* **46:** 1727–1734.

Jain M, Cook GM, Davis FG, Grace MG, Howe GR, Miller AB (1980). A case control study of diet and colorectal cancer. *Int J Cancer* **26:** 757–768.

Jensen OM (1979). Cancer morbidity and causes of death among Danish brewery workers. *Int J Cancer* **23:** 454–463.

Jensen OM (1983). Cancer risk among Danish male Seventh Day Adventists and other temperance society members. *JNCI* **70:** 1011-1014.

Jensen OM, MacLennan R, Warhendorf J (1982). Diet, bowel function, fecal characteristics, and large bowel cancer in Denmark and Finland, *Nutr Cancer* **4:** 5–19.

Kabat GC, Howson CP, Wynder EL (1986). Beer consumption and rectal cancer. *Int J Epidemiol* **15:** 494–501.

Kikendall JW, Bowden PE, Burgess MB, Magnetti C, Woodward J, Langenberg P (1989). Cigarettes and alcohol as independent risk factors for colonic adenomas. *Gastroenterology* **97:** 660–664.

Klatsky AL, Armstrong MA, Friedman GD, Hiatt RA (1988). The relations of alcoholic beverage use to colon and rectal cancer. *Am J Epidemiol* **128:** 1007–1015.

Klurfeld DM (1987). The role of dietary fiber in gastrointestinal diseases. *J Am Diet Assoc* **87:** 1172–1177.

Klurfeld DM, Weber MM, Buck CL, Krichevsky D (1986). Dose-response of colonic carcinogenesis to different amounts and types of cellulose. *Fed Proc* **45:** 1076.

Kono S, Ikeda N, Yanai F, Schinchi D, Imanishi K (1990). Alcoholic beverages and adenomatous polyps of the sigmoid colon: a study of male self-defence officials in Japan. *Int J Epidemiol* **19:** 848–852.

Kune S, Kune GA, Watson LF (1987). Case-control study of dietary etiological factors: the Melbourne colorectal cancer study. *Nutr Cancer* **7:** 21–42.

Kune GA, Kune S, Watson LF (1990). Body weight and physical activity as predictors of colorectal cancer risk. *Nutr Cancer* **13:** 9–17.

La Vecchia C, Negri E, Decarli A, D'Avanzo B, Gallotti L, Gentile A, Franceschi S (1988). A case-control study of diet and colorectal cancer in northern Italy. *Int J Cancer* **41:** 492–498.

Lee HP, Gourley L, Duffy SW, Esteve J, Lee J, Day NE (1989). Colorectal cancer and diet in an Asian population – a case-control study among Singapore Chinese. *Int J Cancer* **43:** 1007-1016.

Lipkin M, Newmark H (1985). Effect of added dietary calcium on colonic epithelial-cell proliferation in subjects at high risk of familial colonic cancer. *N Engl J Med* **313** 1381–1384.

Locke BF, King H (1980). Cancer mortality risk among Japanese in the United States. *JNCI* **65:** 1149–1156.

Lyon JL, Mahoney AW, West DW (1987). Total food intake: a risk factor in colorectal cancer. *JNCI* **78:** 853–861.

MacKeon-Eyssen GE, Bright-See E (1984). Dietary factors in colon cancer: international relationships. *Nutr Cancer* **6:** 160–170.

MacLennan R, Jensen OM, Mosbech J, Vuori H (1978). Diet, transit time, stool weight and colon cancer in two Scandinavian populations. *Am J Clin Nutr* **31:** 5239–5242.

Macquart-Moulin G, Riboli E, Cornee J, Charnay B, Berthezene P, Day N (1986). Case-control study on colorectal cancer and diet in Marseilles. *Int J Cancer* **38:** 183–191.

Macquart-Moulin G, Riboli E, Cornee J, Kaaks R, Berthezene P (1987). Colorectal polyps and diet: a case-control study in Marseilles. *Int J Cancer* **40:** 179–188.

Manousos O, Day NE, Trichopoulos D, Gerovassilis F, Tzonou A, Polychronopoulou A (1983). Diet and colorectal cancer: a case control study in Greece. *Int J Cancer* **32:** 1–5.

Martinez I, Torres R, Frias Z, Colon JR, Fernandez N (1981). Factors associated with adenocarcinomas of the large bowel in Puerto Rico. *Rev Latinoam Oncol Clin* **13:** 13–20.

Mettlin CJ, Schoenfeld ER, Natarajan N (1990). Patterns of milk consumption and risk of cancer. *Nutr Cancer* **13:** 89–99.

Miller AB, Howe GR, Jain M, Craib KJP, Harrison L (1983). Food items and food groups as risk factors in a case control study of diet and colo-rectal cancer. *Int J Cancer* **32:** 155–161.

Modan B, Barrel V, Lubin F, Modan M, Greenberg RA, Graham S (1975). Low Fiber intake as an etiologic factor in cancer of the colon. *JNCI* **55:** 15–18.

Muir C, Waterhouse J, Mack T, Whelan S (1987). Cancer incidence in five continents, Vol IV, IARC Sci Publ No 88, Lyon.

Nauss KM, Locnishar M, Newberne PM (1983). Effect of alterations in the quality and quantity of dietary fat on 1,2-dimethylhydrazine induced colon tumorigenesis in rats. *Cancer Res* **43:** 4083–4090.

Nauss KM, Locnishar M, Sondergaard D, Newberne PM (1984). Lack of effect of dietary fat on N-nitrosomethylurea induced colon tumorigenesis in rats. *Carcinogenesis* **5:** 255–260.

Negri E, La Vecchia C, D'Avanzo B, Franceschi S (1990). Calcium, dairy products and colorectal cancer. *Nutr Cancer* **13:** 255–262.

Neugut AI, Johnsen CM, Forde KA, Treat MR, Nims C (1988).Vitamin supplements among women with adenomatous polyps and cancer of the colon: preliminary findings. *Dis Colon Rectum* **31:** 430–432.

Nigro ND, Bull AW, Klopfer BA, Pak MS, Campbell RL (1979). Effect of dietary fiber on azoxymethane-induced intestinal carcinogenesis in rats. *JNCI* **62:** 1097–1102.

Owen RW, Thompson MH, Hill MJ, Wilpart M, Mainguet P, Roberfroid M (1987). Importance of the ratio of lithocholic acid to deoxycholic acid in large bowel carcinogenesis. *Nutr Cancer* **9:** 67–71.

Philips RL (1975). Role of life style and dietary habits in risk of cancer among Seventh Day Adventists. *Cancer Res* **35:** 3513-3522.

Philips RL (1985). Dietary relationship with fatal colorectal cancer among Seventh-Day Adventist. *JNCI* **74:** 307–317.

Philips RL, Snowdon DA (1983). Association of meat and coffee use with cancers of the large bowel, breast, and prostate among Seventh-Day Adventists: preliminary results. *Cancer Res* **43:** 2403–2408.

Pickle LW, Green E, Ziegler RG, Toledo A, Hoover R, Lynch HT, Fraumeni JF (1984). Colorectal cancer in rural Nebraska. *Cancer Res* **44:** 363–369.

Pollack ES, Nomura AMY, Heilbrun LK, Stemmermann GN, Green SB (1984). Prospective alcohol consumption and cancer. *New Engl J Med* **310:** 617–621.

Potter JD, MacMichael AJ, Hartshorne JM (1982). Alcohol and beer consumption in relation to cancers of the bowel and lung: an extended correlation analysis. *J Chronic Dis* **35:** 833–842.

Potter JD, MacMichael AJ (1986). Diet and cancer of the colon and rectum. A case control study. *JNCI* **76:** 557–569.

Prizont R (1987). Absence of large bowel tumors in rats injected with 1,2 dimethylhydrazine and fed high dietary cellulose. *Dig Dis Sci* **32:** 1418–1421.

Reddy BS, Narisawa T, Weisburger JH (1976). Effect of a diet with high levels of protein and fat on colon carcinogenesis in F 344 rats treated with 1,2-dimethylhydrazine. *JNCI* **57:** 567–569.

Reddy BS, Watanabe K, Weisburger JH (1977). Effect of a high fat diet on colon carcinogenesis in F 344 rats treated wtih 1,2-dimethyl hydrazine, methylazoxymethanol acetate or methylonitrosourea. *Cancer Res* **37:** 4156–4159.

Reddy BS, Hirot AN (1979). Effect of dietary ascorbic acid on 1-2 dimethyl-hydrazine induced colon cancer in rats. *Fed Proc* **38:** 714–716.

Reddy BS, Mori H (1981). Effect of dietary wheat bran and dehydrated citrus fiber on 3,2-dimethyl-4-aminobiphenyl-induced intestinal carcinogenesis in F344 rats. *Carcinogenesis* **2:** 21–25.

Reddy BS, Mori H, Nicolais N (1981). Effect of dietary wheat bran and dehydrated citrus fiber on azoxymethane-induced intestinal carcinogenesis in Fischer 344 rats. *JNCI* **66**: 553–557.

Reddy BS, Maeura Y, Wayman M (1983). Effect of dietary corn bran and autohydrolyzed lignin on 3,2-dimethyl-4-aminobiphenyl-induced intestinal carcinogenesis in male F344 rats. *JNCI* **71**: 419–423.

Reddy BS, Tanaka T, Simi B (1985). Effect of different levels of dietary trans fat or corn oil on azoxymethane-induced. Colon carcinogenesis in F 344 rats. *JNCI* **75**: 791–798.

Riboli E (1986). In Muir CS, Wagner G eds. Directory of ongoing research in cancer epidemiology. IARC Sci Publ No 80, Lyon p109.

Rosenberg L, Werler MM, Palmer JR, Daufman DW, Warshauer ME, Stolley PD, Shapiro S (1989). The risks of cancers of the colon and rectum in relation to coffee consumption. *Am J Epidemiol* **130**: 895–903.

Rozen P, Fireman Z, Fine N, Wax Y, Ron E (1989). Oral calcium suppresses increased rectal epithelial proliferation of persons at risk of colorectal cancer. *Gut* **30**: 650–655.

Slattery ML, Sorenson W, Ford MH (1988). Dietary calcium intake as a mitigating factor in colon cancer. *Am J Epidemiol* **128**: 504-514.

Stemmermann GN, Normura AMY, Heilbrun LK (1984). Dietary fat and the risk of colorectal cancer. *Cancer Res* **44**: 4633–4637.

Stemmermann GN, Nomura AM, Chyou PH, Yoshizawa C (1990). Prospective study of alcohol intake and large bowel cancer. *Dig Dis and Sciences* **35**: 1414–1420.

Thornton JR (1981). High colonic pH promotes colorectal cancer. *Lancet* **1**: 1081–1082.

Trudel JL, Senterman MK, Borwn RA (1983). The fat/fiber antagonism in experimental colon carcinogenesis. *Surgery* **94**: 691–696.

Tuyns AJ, Pequignot G, Gignoux M, Valla A (1982). Cancer of the digestive tract, alcohol and tobacco. *Int J Cancer* **30**: 9–11.

Tuyns AJ, Haelterman M, Kaaks R (1987). Colorectal cancer and the intake of nutrients: oligosaccharides are a risk factor, fats are not. A case-control study in Belgium. *Nutr Cancer* **10**: 185-196.

Tuyns AJ, Kaaks R, Haelterman M (1988). Colorectal cancer and the consumption of foods: a case-control study in Belgium. *Nutr Cancer* **11**: 189–204.

Ward JM, Yamamoto RS, Weisburger JH (1973). Cellulose dietary bulk and azoxymethane-induced intestinal cancer. *JNCI* **51**: 713-715.

Watanabe K, Reddy BS, Weisburger JH, Krichevsky D (1979). Effect of dietary alfalfa, pectin and wheat bran on azoxymethane- or methylnitrosourea-induced colon carcinogenesis in F344 rats. *JNCI* **63**: 141–145.

West DW, Slattery ML, Robinson LM, Schuman KL, Ford MH, Mahoney AW, Lyon JL, Sorensen AW (1989). Dietary intake and colon cancer: sex- and anatomic site-specific associations. *Am J Epidemiol* **130**: 883–894.

Willett WC, Stampfer MJ, Colditz GA, Rosner BA, Speizer FE (1990). Relation of meat, fat and fiber intake to the risk of colon cancer in a prospective study among women. *New Eng J Med* **323**: 1664–1672.

Wilpart M (1987). Dietary fat and fibre and experimental colon carcinogenesis: a critical review of published evidence. In Causation and prevention of colorectal cancer. Faire J, Hill MJ eds. Elsevier, Amsterdam pp. 85–98.

Wilpart M, Roberfroid M (1987). Intestinal carcinogenesis and dietary fibers: the influence of cellulose or fybogel chronically given after exposure to DMH. *Nutr Cancer* **10:** 39–51.

Wilson RB, Hutcheson DP, Widemanf V (1977). Dimethylhydrazine induced colon tumors in rats fed diets containing beef fat or corn oil with and without wheat bran. *Am J Clin Nutr* **30:** 176-181.

Young TB, Wolf DA (1988). Case-control study of proximal and distal colon cancer and diet in Wisconsin. *Int J Cancer* **43:** 167-175.

CHAPTER 7

Diet and Breast Cancer

F DE WAARD

Department of Epidemiology
University of Utrecht, The Netherlands

Large differences in breast cancer incidence between countries suggest that the environment in which we live has a profound influence on the breast. The pattern of incidence is rather similar to that of colon cancer in the sense that affluence and the life-style which is prevalent in the "Western" world seems to enhance risk.

Both reproduction and nutrition are thought to be involved in the aetiology of breast cancer. Concerning nutrition international correlation studies focussed on the relationship between breast cancer incidence or mortality and the per capita intake of dietary fat, in particular animal fat (Carroll, 1975). Although the weaknesses of drawing causal inferences from ecological correlations are well-known, the said relationship apparently has had a strong appeal to the scientific community. Case-control studies have provided modest support for a relation with dietary fat but cohort studies do not confirm this (Prentice *et al.*, 1989).

Evidence of a genuine relation has been strengthened by experiments in rodents. The pioneer studies by Tannenbaum *et al.* (1945) in the 1940's which had almost been forgotten, were revived by Carroll (1975) in Canada and several others in the United States. Considering mechanisms two hypotheses were advanced: one pointing to the high energy content of fat and the other suggesting a specific effect of various dietary fats: saturated as well as mono- or polyunsaturated fats (Cohen, 1981).

I have a preference for the high energy hypothesis not only because of the new insight on energy provided by fats (Pariza, 1987) and the convincing animal experiments by Kritchevsky *et al.* (1984) but also because in human endocrinology there are well-established links between symptoms of over nutrition and steroid hormone metabolism.

In the 1960's we advanced the hypothesis that overweight was associated with breast cancer through increased oestrogen production of extra-ovarian origin in postmenopausal women (De Waard *et al.*, 1964, 1969). This finding was confirmed by other authors (though not all of them) and

69

present-day insight seems to point to its role in enhancing growth of existing breast cancer; after diagnosis this boils down to obesity being an unfavourable prognostic factor (Newman *et al.*, 1986).

Our original idea that obesity would be able to explain most of the international variation of breast cancer incidence began to waver because of some new observations made by ourselves as well as by others. In a prospective study we found that body height was as important as body weight (De Waard *et al.*, 1974) and MacMahon immediately pointed out that apparently events occurring during adolescence were involved in determining risk (MacMahon, 1975).

A time-trend study in Iceland (Bjarnason *et al.*, 1974) and migrant studies of Japanese to the United States (Dunn, 1975) strongly suggested that increases in incidence over time take place birth cohort-wise; adaptation to the new environment had to occur at an early age in order to bring about a high breast cancer risk (De Waard, 1978).This notion combined with the knowledge about the risk factors occurring at a relatively young age (such as age at menarche, body height, age at first full-time pregnancy) has enriched our insight into the aetiology of human breast cancer. Both age at menarche and body height are clearly related to nutrition: in affluent societies women have on average an early menarche and they are tall (Tanner, 1962).

In the context of the present Symposium it is not possible to describe all the considerations leading to the concept that the period in a women's life between the beginning of breast development (thelarche, which slightly precedes menarche) and the first full-time pregnancy is of major importance in determining breast cancer risk. In societies where girls experience menarche early (due to rich nutrition) it can be inferred from studies by MacMahon *et al.* (1982) and Apter *et al.* (1989) that oestrogen production during adolescence is higher than in societies with on average a later menarche. This tends to increase proliferation of breast epithelia.

As long as there is a delay in becoming pregnant proliferation goes on unabated. In the same societies where proliferation begins early and at an increased pace there is a larger time delay before the first child is born. This is an undesirable trend. Through the work of the Russo *et al.* (1982) we now understand that the hormones of pregnancy bring about differentiation of breast epithelia which renders them resistant to carcinogenesis.

Evidence is accumulating that indeed in the adolescent breast before the first priming for motherhood (differentiation, needed for lactation) atypical lobules called ALA by Wellings (1975) are being formed (De Waard and Trichopoulos, 1988). Their number is likely to be determined by the proliferation rate during those years which in turn depends on oestrogen levels. These levels (like menarche) are determined by nutritional factors.

According to this hypothesis an important nutritional factor in the aetiology of breast cancer is (or are) the same as those responsible for early menarche and tall height. If this hypothesis is correct the period of life suitable for preventive action should be adolescence and early adulthood. This implies that the large and expensive American nutrition intervention study called the Women's Health Trial (Greenwald, 1988) might hit at the wrong target since it aims at reducing the consumption of dietary fat in women aged 40–50.

Which *recommendations* can be made based on present-day knowledge?

A. Recommendations for Research

1.   Non-invasive methods for study of the adolescent female breast should be developed. Magnetic resonance spectroscopy (Merchant *et al.*, 1988) might be an important tool.

2.   The effect of weight reduction on the prognosis of breast cancer in obese postmenopausal women should be studied in a randomised trial. In a feasibility study (to be published) we tend to conclude that with intensive dietary guidance an average weight loss of 7 kg can be achieved over a period of 2–3 years.

B. Recommendations to the Public:

No specific recommendations as to nutritional options for preventing the occurrence of breast cancers are to be made. Certainly, being moderate in food consumption and having physical exercise regularly is part of a healthy life-style generally; monitoring body weight during adolescence and postmenopausal years may be relevant for breast cancer occurrence.

C. Recommendations for the Food Market:

These are as general as those directed to the public. The concept of balanced food eaten with moderation should be stressed.

Summary

A selected menu from the vast literature on nutrition and breast cancer is served. Attention is drawn to nutritional factors operating early in life which modify the "milieu interieur".

Doubts are expressed as to the potential success of the Women's Health Trial to be undertaken in the United States.

A randomised trial of weight reduction concerning the prognosis of breast cancer in obese postmenopausal women should be considered.

References

Apter D, Reinila M, Vikho R (1989). Some endocrine characteristics of early menarche, a risk factor for breast cancer, are preserved into adulthood. *Int J Cancer* **44:** 783–7.

Bjarnason O, Day NE, Snaedal G, Tulinius H (1974). The effect of year of birth on the breast cancer age-incidence curve in Iceland. *Int J Cancer* **13:** 689–96.

Carroll KK (1975). Experimental evidence of dietary factors and hormone-dependent cancers. *Cancer Res* **35:** 3374–83.

Cohen LA (1981). Mechanisms by which dietary fat may stimulate mammary carcinogenesis in experimental animals. *Cancer Res* **41:** 3808–10.

De Waard F, Baanders-van Halewijn EA, Huizinga J (1964). The biomodal age distribution of patients with mammary carcinoma. *Cancer* **17:** 141–51.

De Waard F, Baanders-van Halewijn EA (1969). Cross-sectional data on estrogenic smears in a postmenopausal population. *Acta Cytol (Phylad)* **13:** 675–8.

De Waard F, Baanders-van Halewijn EA (1974). A prospective study in general practice on breast cancer risk in postmenopausal women. *Int J Cancer* **14:** 153–60.

De Waard F (1978). Recent time trends in breast cancer incidence. *Prev Med* **7:** 160–7.

De Waard F, Trichopoulos D (1988). A unifying concept of the aetiology of human breast cancer. *Int J Cancer* **41:** 666–9.

Dunn JE (1975). Cancer epidemiology in populations of the United States – with emphasis on Hawaii and California – and Japan. *Cancer Res* **35:** 3240–5.

Greenwald P (1988). Issues raised by The Women's Health Trial. *JNCI* **80:** 788–90.

Kritchevsky D, Weber MM, Klurfeld DM (1984). Dietary fat versus caloric content. Initiation and promotion of DMBA-induced mammary tumorigenesis in rats. *Cancer Res* **44:** 3174–7.

MacMahon B (1975). Formal discussion of De Waard's paper. *Cancer Res* **35:** 3357–58.

MacMahon B, Trichopoulos D, Brown J *et al.* (1982). Age at menarche, urine estrogens and breast cancer risk. *Int J Cancer* **30:** 427–31.

Merchant TE, Gierke LW, Meneses P, Glonek T (1988). 31P Magnetic resonance spectroscopic profiles of neoplastic human breast tissues. *Cancer Res* **48:** 5112–8.

Newman SC, Miller AB, Howe ER (1986). A study of the effect of weight and dietary fat on breast cancer survival time. *Amer J Epidemiol* **123:** 767–74.

Pariza MW (1987). Fat, calories and mammary carcinogenesis: net energy effects. *Amer J Clin Nutr* **45:** 261–3.

Prentice RL, Pepe M, Self SG (1989). Dietary fat and breast cancer: a quantitative assessment of the epidemiological literature and a discussion of methodological issues. *Cancer Res* **49:** 3147–56.

Russo J, Tay LK, Russo IH (1982). Differentiation of the mammary gland and susceptibility to carcinogenesis. *Breast Cancer Res Treat* **2:** 5–73.

Tannenbaum A (1945). The genesis and growth of tumors. II. Effect of caloric restriction *per se*. *Cancer Res* **5:** 615–25.

Tanner JM (1962). Growth at adolescence; Blackwell Scient Publ.

Wellings SR, Jensen HM, Marcum RS (1975). An atlas of subgross pathology of the human breast with special reference to possible precancerous lesions. *JNCI* **55:** 231–73.

CHAPTER 8

Diet and Gastric Cancer

PI REED

Lady Sobell Gastrointestinal Unit, Wexham Park Hospital,
Slough, Berks, SL2 4HL, UK

Although the causation of gastric cancer (GC) is complex and multifactorial the role of diet as a modulator of GC incidence has received wide recognition in recent years in the light of the progressive reduction of this cancer during the past four decades. Numerically it is still the second most common cancer world-wide and in many developing countries the most common. Thus the magnitude of the problem varies with the degree of development – overall in developing countries GC ranks second after cervical cancer, while in developed countries it ranks fourth after lung, colorectal and breast cancer. There are large differences in incidence among populations, with a 2–3 fold excess in males and it increases with age in both sexes. An inverse socioeconomic as well as a North-South geographical gradient have been observed in most populations in the Northern hemisphere (Muir *et al.*, 1987). An increased risk has been linked to certain occupations including coal mining, fishing and agriculture, and since occupations are clearly linked to socioeconomic status some of the observed excess risk might be attributable to dietary habits. The gradual decline in GC in many populations may be a reflection of the improving economic conditions (Hirayama, 1980). Epidemiological studies in migrants in the USA have also greatly helped in our understanding of the dynamics of GC and its precursor lesions. Migrants from high risk areas such as Japan moving to low risk areas such as Hawaii and California were shown to retain the high risk for the disease unless they migrated in childhood or early adult life (Hill, 1990). It is probable that these differences are related to a change in diet. These and other published studies have provided convincing evidence of the critical importance of exposure in early life in determining the risk of developing, as a first stage, the precancerous lesions and later GC itself.

   Extensive epidemiological studies in Japan, which until recently had the highest GC incidence in the world, have highlighted the importance of diet and nutrition in GC incidence (Hirayama, 1988). The Japanese National

Nutritional Survey demonstrated that striking changes had taken place in the Japanese diet following World War 2. For instance, between 1949 and 1978 there was a 28-fold increase in the consumption of milk and milk products and the ratios of increases in other food items were notable for meat 12.8, eggs 13.0, oil 10.2, fruit 6.6. The decreasing ratio in the age adjusted death rate for GC in 12 districts in Japan correlated closely with fat and vitamin A intake. In another prospective study of 265,118 adults aged 40 or over, during the period 1966–1978, a significant inverse trend between GC incidence and intake of green-yellow vegetables was demonstrated both in males and females and smokers and non-smokers (Hirayama *et al.*, 1985).

The description of 2 major histological types of GC (Lauren, 1965), the diffuse and intestinal and subsequent studies by Lehtola (1978) led to a clearer understanding of the epidemiological aspects. It is the incidence of the intestinal type of GC, found predominantly in the antrum and body of the stomach, which has been decreasing steadily, whereas the incidence of the diffuse type, evenly divided between the sexes and occurring anywhere in the stomach which has remained relatively constant in all populations over the years.

Correa *et al.* (1975) proposed a model for intestinal type gastric carcino-genesis suggesting a multistage process probably initiated early in life and starting with multifocal chronic atrophic gastritis progressing to intestinal metaplasia (IM) then to epithelial dysplasia and ultimately GC. In the light of increasing knowledge obtained from multidisciplinary research this model has undergone several revisions (Charnley *et al.*, 1982; Correa *et al.*, 1988; Correa, 1991). In this model (Figure 1) it was proposed that the reduction of nitrate (NO_3) to nitrite (NO_2) through the action of nitrate-reducing bacteria in the saliva and in an hypoacidic stomach could result in the subsequent formation of *N*-nitroso compounds (NOC) which could act as promoters during the later stage of carcinogenesis and that their effects could also be modified by a number of environmental factors. However, the endogenous formation of NOC is not confined to bacterial action alone, either through chemical nitrosation with bacterially formed NO_2 or by bacteria themselves, since *N*-nitrosation may also occur under normal gastric (acidic) conditions. This has been convincingly confirmed *in vivo* in man by Ohshima and Bartsch (1981) who showed that *N*-nitro-soproline is formed in the stomach following the ingestion of proline and NO_3 and excreted in the urine in inverse ratio to gastric pH, this reaction being maximal at pH and which can be inhibited by vitamin C, a potent antioxidant. *N*-Nitroso compounds, several hundred of which have now been identified and many of which are either carcinogenic or mutagenic, have been shown to be carcinogenic in all 40 animal species tested and it is unlikely that *Homo sapiens* would be an exception (Bogovski and Bogovski, 1981; Schmdhl and Scherf, 1984).

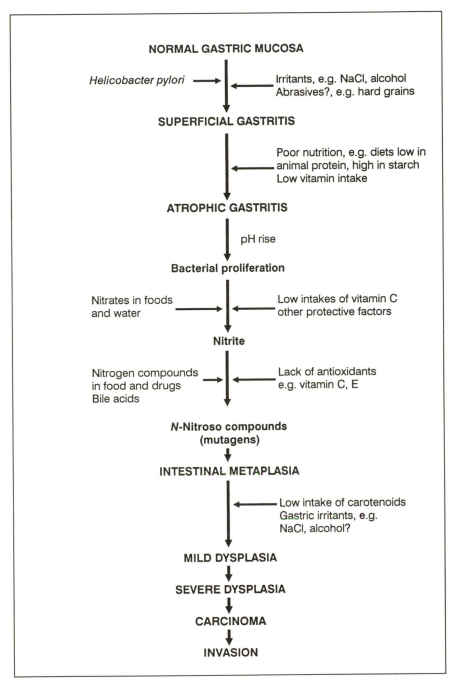

Figure 1 A model for gastric carcinogenesis (After Correa, 1988)

To test the importance of the role of NO_3 numerous epidemiological studies have made correlations between NO_3 exposure and GC risk and their results have been reviewed (Hill, 1988). While the majority have demonstrated a positive association, some studies have contradicted the earlier hypothesis that a high exogenous NO_3 exposure increases the GC risk (Forman *et al.*, 1985). The evidence for and against this view has been reviewed by Preussmann and Tricker (1988). It should be noted that while NO_3 *per se* does not constitute a cancer risk, it acts as a precursor to NO_2, a very reactive molecule capable of nitrating other nitrogen containing substrates formed in the body by bacterial reduction, and which reacts directly or indirectly to produce NOC. Thus the nitrate burden should be regarded as an "indirect risk" factor and NOC formation as a "direct risk" factor in human carcinogenesis. The importance of dietary factors, particularly vegetables, has been highlighted by two epidemiological studies in the Far East. In China the NO_3 and NO_2 burden from vegetables and drinking water was shown to be higher in an high risk area for GC (Xu, 1981) and higher salivary and gastric juice NO_3 and NO_2 levels were also demonstrated in fasting patients with chronic gastritis. In the second study from Japan (Hirayama, 1988), the NO_3 burden, as determined by its urinary excretion, was higher in the low GC risk area and correlated well with vegetable consumption. Moreover, the dietary NO_3 content depends also on the form in which the vegetables are eaten. Pickled vegetables often have much higher NO_3 levels than if they are raw. This would suggest that the diet and dietary sources of NO_3 may be more significant than the total NO_3 burden. The presence of *N*-nitrosation inhibitors, such as vitamin C and phenolic compounds, in vegetables and their ability to reduce endogenous N-nitrosation, and thereby the GC risk, in low risk populations which show high salivary NO_3 levels, may also be relevant. Large variations in the intake of NO_3 both within and between populations were confirmed in a recent ECP-Intersalt collaborative study of 24 hour urinary NO_3 excretion in 5,700 subjects in 48 populations from 28 countries (Hill, personal communication). This was due, in part to the type of diet, notably its vegetable content. NO_3 excretion was also found to he higher in low income populations, e.g. parts of Mexico and Eastern Europe, in the age group 20–29 years. In Colombia NO_3 ingestion and urinary output have been correlated with gastric precancerous lesions (Correa, 1983). On the other hand, in England, where NO_3 is mostly obtained from fresh vegetables, Forman *et al.* (1985) found an inverse correlation between NO_3 intake and urinary levels and GC risk. It has also been shown that NO_3 intake results in excessive gastric NO_2 only in subjects with chronic atrophic gastritis (Eisenbrand *et al.*, 1984). A review of all available data would indicate that in developed countries there is only weak evidence for dietary NO_3 involvement in GC development, whereas in developing countries, such as China and Colombia, the situation is more complex in view of the high incidence of gastric hypoacidity and dietary deficiencies and a high NO_3 burden may thus be but one of several factors responsible for the higher GC incidence.

The role of amine precursors to NOC relevant to human GC induction has been studied also in various countries, again with conflicting results, and the lack of knowledge about specific amine precursors to potentially relevant gastric carcinogens is a major gap in our understanding of human gastric cancer formation. Positive epidemiological studies have emphasised the nutritional status and specific food items. For instance, smoked fish has been positively associated with GC risk in Iceland (Dungal, 1985), Japan (Hitchcock and Scheiner, 1965) and Norway (Bjelke, 1974) but not in Colombia (Correa *et al.*, 1983). Also following nitrosation, a common fish constituent of the Japanese diet was shown to induce adenocarcinoma in the glandular stomach of experimental rats (Weisburger *et al.*, 1980). Sun-dried herrings and sardines were shown to have strong mutagenic activity after NO_2 treatment (Wakabayashi *et al.*, 1985).

Epidemiological data from Colombia have shown an high intake of fava beans in high GC risk populations (Correa *et al.*, 1983). A very potent mutagen, whose precursor was identified as 4-chloro-6-methoxyindole, is produced following nitrosation of fava beans (Yang *et al.*, 1984). Other observations suggest that dietary substituted indoles, widely abundant in green plants of the brassica family, could also react with NO_2 in the human stomach resulting in DNA damage (Wakabayashi *et al.*, 1985).

Dry heating (pyrolysis) of food products rich in amino acids and proteins produces highly mutagenic aromatic amine compounds (Huber and Lutz, 1984). Certain Japanese foods, including grilled beef, chicken and onions and boiled dried fish have been shown to contain between 1 and 650 $\mu g/kg$ of pyrolysis products, and the most important representatives of this group of compounds have been shown to be carcinogenic in several animal species (Ochiai *et al.*, 1984). Thus in the presence of nitrosatable amine precursors the potential formation of NOC and/or alkylating species, which may be relevant for GC induction, remains a plausible working hypothesis. However, the occurrence and nature of nitrosatable amines in the human stomach remains one of the major missing links in our knowledge about human endogenous NOC formation.

Another factor related to diet thought to have made a large impact on GC incidence is the introduction of refrigeration. There has been a consistent relationship between the start of the decrease in the incidence of GC and the use of refrigeration using ice-boxes, refrigerators and deep-freezes in Japan (Hirayama, 1980) and Spain (Grens *et al.*, 1991). Refrigeration makes the use of salt as a food preservative redundant thus further reducing the risk of GC and also decreasing the likelihood of growth of moulds in foods (Joosens and Kesteloot, 1988). Furthermore, salt itself has been suggested as being associated with GC (Joosens and

Geboers, 1981). Excessive use of salt induces gastritis (Kodama *et al.*, 1984) and in experimental animals this has been shown to be accompanied by markedly increased cell replication, a critical event in carcinogenesis (Charnley and Tannenbaum, 1985). Several case-control studies, although fairly subjective, have shown remarkable consistency indicating that heavy use of salt would be compatible with a 50% increase in GC risk.

The role of micronutrients and vitamins as inhibitors of *N*-nitrosation in the aetiology of GC has also been widely studied. That vegetable consumption does have a protective effect on GC risk has been well documented (Graham *et al.*, 1972; Hu *et al.*, 1988; Jedrychowski *et al.*, 1986; La Vecchia *et al.*, 1987; Risch *et al*, 1985; Trichopoulos *et al.*, 1985; Forman, 1991). This effect has been demonstrated either in developing countries or high risk areas. However one case control study in the UK (Acheson and Doll, 1964) failed to show any effect of vegetable consumption on GC risk. A protective effect on GC risk has also been shown for fruit (Forman, 1991). A prospective study of the association between vitamins A, C, E and carotene and subsequent risk of overall, lung, stomach and gastro-intestinal cancer mortality of 2,974 men in Basle, Switzerland revealed that plasma vitamin A levels were significantly lower in men who subsequently died of stomach cancer. The authors also suggested a new parameter called the normative cumulative index which sums the antioxidant vitamins A, C and β-carotene and when age-standardised was shown to be significantly depressed for all major cancer types (Gey *et al*, 1987). These findings were confirmed by a recent updated analysis at a 12 year follow up which found that stomach and lung cancer were associated with significantly lower mean plasma carotene levels and men who subsequently developed stomach cancer also had lower mean vitamin C and lipid adjusted vitamin A levels than survivors (Eichholzer-Helbling and Stdhelin *et al.*, 1991).

In 1985 the ECP-EURONUT intestinal metaplasia (IM) study was initiated (West *et al.*, 1988) with the aim of studying the early stages of the development of the intestinal type of GC with special reference to dietary factors. Preliminary results have been published (Reed, 1990) and in summary have shown that patients with intestinal metaplasia (IM) in the UK have a lower intake of foods rich in antioxidant vitamins compared with controls with histologically normal stomachs and controls without upper-gastrointestinal symptoms. This was accompanied by lower serum vitamin C levels in the IM patient group. Serum selenium concentrations were not significantly different between the IM and control patients (UK Subgroup, ECP Study Group, 1991). The patients recruited to this study are to be re-endoscoped and biopsied 5 years after the entry endoscopy to establish whether changes in the gastric histopathology have taken place and relate any changes noted to the diet and vitamin levels at entry into the study.

From the results of these and other studies it seemed logical to move to the use of micronutrients and vitamins in planned intervention in populations at increased risk of GC.

To date only a few very limited intervention studies have been carried out in patients at increased risk of developing GC. The treatment period has been short, patient numbers small and results equivocal. The data from only two have been reported but other studies are either being planned or are already in progress. We studied the effect of vitamin C administration in patients who had undergone gastric surgery for benign peptic ulcer disease (Reed *et al.*, 1989) and demonstrated a significant reduction in mean NO_2 and NOC concentrations in fasting gastric juice after 4 weeks treatment with 4 g vitamin C daily, this reduction being most marked in patients with partial gastrectomy. Krytopoulos (1984) showed that supplementation of the normal diet of subjects with 400 mg daily each of vitamin C and α-tocopherol resulted in a significant reduction in the mutagenic compounds excreted with faeces suggesting that antioxidants in the diet may have a role in lowering the body's exposure to endogenously formed mutagens. In a third study Correa (personal communication) not unexpectedly was unable to show any effect on gastric histology in 60 patients with atrophic gastritis after 2 months treatment with either vitamins A, C or E compared to placebo.

Although the wealth of available epidemiological case-control and preliminary interventional study data have clearly established the dietary impact on GC risk, there is no doubt that the development of GC is multifactorial (Correa, 1991). It is now possible to identify at least three factors which probably play a significant role in increasing the GC risk, two of which are dietary, excessive salt intake and a low intake of fresh fruit and vegetables, and the third is *Helicobacter pylori* infection (Parsonnet *et al.*, 1991; Nomura *et al.*, 1991). Thus the diet of populations at high risk of GC is characterised by a low intake of animal fats and proteins, high intakes of starches and carbohydrates (mainly from grains and starchy roots), high salt ingestion, high dietary nitrate intakes (from water and foodstuffs) with low intakes of fresh fruit and raw vegetables and salads. We await the outcome of future studies which, hopefully, will confirm that minimizing these risk factors, especially in high risk areas, will lead to further progressive reduction in the intestinal type GC incidence world wide.

Acknowledgements

I wish to thank Belinda Johnston for her valuable contribution to our studies on GC and assistance in preparation of this manuscript, Dr Michael Hill for a long standing fruitful and continuing collaboration and many helpful comments and the Cancer Research Campaign for supporting one of the studies referred to in the text.

References

Muir C, Waterhouse J, Mack T, Powell J, Whelan S (eds) (1987). Cancer incidence in Five Continents, Vol V, IARC Sci Publ No 75, Lyon, IARC,

Hirayama T (1980). Changing patterns in the incidence of gastric cancer. In *Gastric Cancer* (eds Fielding JWl, Newman CE, Ford CHJ, Jones BG); Pergamon Press, Oxford, pp 1–16.

Hill MJ (1990). Epidemiology and mechanism of gastric carcinogenesis. In *New Trends in Gastric Cancer: Background and Videosurgery* (eds Reed PI, Carboni M, Johnston BJ, Guadagni S); Kluwer Academic Publishers, Dordrecht/Boston/London, pp 3–12.

Hirayama T (1988). Actions suggested by gastric cancer epidemiological studies in Japan. In *Gastric carcinogenesis* (eds Reed PI, Hill MJ); Excerpta Medica, Amsterdam, pp 209–27.

Hirayama T (1985). Diet and cancer: feasibility and importance of prospective cohort study. In *Diet and Human Carcinogenesis, International Congress Series 685* (eds Joosens JV, Hill MJ, Geboers J); Excerpta Medica, Amsterdam, pp 191–8.

Correa P, Haenszel W, Cuello C, Tannenbaum S, Archer M (1975). A model for gastric cancer epidemiology. *Lancet* ii: 58–60.

Charnley G, Tannenbaum SR, Correa P (1982). Gastric cancer: An etiological model. In *Banbury Report 12, Nitrosamines and Human Cancer* (ed Magee PN); Cold Spring Harbor Laboratory, New York, pp 503–22.

Correa P (1988). A human model of gastric carcinogenesis. *Cancer Res* **48**: 3554.

Correa P (1991). The epidemiology of gastric cancer. *World J Surg* **15**: 228–4.

Lehtola J (1978). Family study of gastric carcinoma; with special reference to histological types. *Scand J Gastroenterol* **13** (**Suppl 50**): 1–54.

Lauren P (1965). The two histological main types of gastric carcinoma: diffuse and so-called intestinal type. *Acta Path Microbiol Scand* **64**: 31–49.

Ohshima H, Bartsch H (1981). Quantitative estimation of endogenous nitrosation in humans by monitoring N-nitrosoproline excreted in the urine. *Cancer Res* **41**: 3658–62.

Bogovski P, Bogovski S (1981). Animal species in which N-nitroso compounds induce cancer. Special report. *Int J Cancer* **27**: 471–4.

Schmahl D, Scherf HR (1984). Carcinogenic activity of N-nitroso-diethylamine in snakes (*Python reticulatus* Biodae). In *N-nitroso compounds: Occurrence, Biological Effects and Relevance to Human Cancer* (eds Bartsch H, O'Neill IK, Von Borstel R, Miller CT, Long J); IARC Scient Publ 57, IARC, Lyon, pp. 677–82.

Hill MJ (1987). Gastric carcinogenesis: Luminal Factors. In *Gastric Carcinogenesis* (eds Reed PI, Hill MJ) Excerpta Medica, Amsterdam, pp 187–200.

Correa P, Cuello C, Fajardo LF (1983). Diet and gastric cancer: Nutrition survey in a high-risk area. *J Natl Cancer Inst* **70**: 673–8.

Forman D, Al-Dabbagh S, Doll R (1985). Nitrates, nitrites and gastric cancer in Great Britain. *Nature* **313**: 620–5.

Preussmann R, Tricker AR (1988). Endogenous nitrosamine formation and nitrate burden in relation to gastric cancer epidemiology. In *Gastric Carcinogenesis* (eds Reed PI, Hill MJ) Excerpta Medica, Amsterdam, pp 147–62.

Xu GW (1981). Gastric Cancer in China: a review. *J Roy Soc Med* **74**: 210–11.

Thaler H (1976). Nitrates and gastric carcinoma. *Deutsch Medizinische Wochenscrift* **101**: 1740–2.

Eisenbrand G, Adam B, Peter M, Malfterheimer P, Schlag P (1984). Formation of nitrite in gastric juice of patients with various gastric disorders after ingestion of standard dose of nitrate. A possible factor in gastric carcinogenesis. Scient Publ No. 57, IARC, Lyon, pp 963–8.

Dungal N (1961). The special problem of stomach cancer in Iceland: with particular reference to dietary factors. *JAMA* **178**: 789–98.

Hitchcock DR, Scheiner SL (1965). The early diagnosis of gastric cancer. *Surg Gynecol Obstet* **113**: 665–72.

Bjelke E (1974). Epidemiologic studies of cancer of the stomach, colon and rectum: with special emphasis on the role of diet. *Scand J Gastroenterol* **9** (**Suppl 31**): 1–235.

Weisburger JH, Marquardt H, Hirota H (1980). Induction of cancer of the glandular stomach by extract of nitrite treated fish. *J Natl Cancer Inst* **64**: 163–7.

Wakabayashi K, Nagao M, Chung TH, Yin M, Karai I, Ochiai M, Tahira T, Sugimura T (1985). Appearance of direct-acting mutagenicity of various foodstuffs produced in Japan and Southeast Asia on nitrite treatment. *Mutat Res* **158**: 119–24.

Yang D, Tannenbaum SR, Bucki B, Lee GCM (1984) 4-chloro-6-methyoxyindole is a precursor of a potent mutagen that forms during nitrosation of the fava beans (Vicia faba). *Carcinogenesis* **5**: 1219–24

Wakabayashi K, Nagao M, Ochiai M, Tahira T, Yamaizumi Z, Sugimura T (1986). A mutagen precursor in Chinese cabbage, indole-3-acetonitrile which becomes mutagenic on nitrite treatment. *Mutat Res* **143**: 17–21.

Huber KW, Lutz WK (1984). Methylation of DNA by incubation with methylamine and nitrite. *Carcinogenesis* **5**: 1729–32

Ochiai M, Wakabayashi K, Nagao M, Sugimura T (1984). Tyramine is a major mutagen precursor in soy sauce, being convertible to a mutagen by nitrite. *Gann* **75**: 1–3.

Greus PC, Vizcaino CC. Sanchez JLA, Piquer DC, Serrulla ST (1991). Levels of household refrigeration of foodstuffs and mortality through stomach cancer in Spain (1960–86). *Europ J Cancer Prevent* **1** (**Suppl 1**): 25–6.

Joosens JV, Kesteloot H (1988). Diet and stomach cancer. In *Gastric Carcinogenesis* (eds Reed PI, Hill MJ). Excerpta Medica Amsterdam, pp 105–26.

Joosens JV, Geboers J (1981). Nutrition and gastric cancer. *Nutr Cancer* **2**: 250–61.

Kodama M, Kodama T, Susuki H, Kondon K (1984). Effect of rice and salty rice diet on the structure of mouse stomach. *Nutr Cancer* **6**: 135–47.

Charnley G, Tannenbaum SR (1985). Flow cytometric analysis of the effect of sodium chloride on gastric cancer risk in the rat. *Cancer Res* **45**: 5608–16.

Graham S, Schotz W, Martino P (1972). Alimentary factors in the epidemiology of gastric cancer. *Cancer* **30**: 927–38.

Hu J, Shang S, Jia E, Wang Q, Liu Y, Wu Y, Cheng Y (1988). Diet and cancer of the stomach: a case-control study in China. *Int J Cancer* **41**: 331–5.

Jedrychowski W, Wahrendorf J, Popiela T, Rachtan J (1986) A case-control study of dietary factors and stomach cancer risk in Poland. *Int J Cancer* **37**: 837–42.

La Vecchia C, Negri E, Decarli A, D'Avanzo B, Franceschi S (1987). A case-control study of diet and gastric cancer in Northern Italy. *Int J Cancer* **40**: 484–9.

Risch HA, Jain M, Choi NW, Fodor JG, Pfeiffer CJ, Howe GR, Harrison LW, Craib

KJP, Miller AB (1985). Dietary factors and the incidence of cancer of the stomach. *Am J Epidemiol* **122:** 947–59.

Trichopoulos D, Ouranos G, Day NE, Tzonou A, Manousos O, Papadimitriou C, Trichopoulos A (1985). Diet and cancer of stomach: a case-control study in Greece. *Int J Cancer* **36:** 291–7.

Acheson ED, Doll R (1964). Dietary factors in carcinoma of the stomach: a study of 100 cases and 200 controls. *Gut* **51:** 126–31.

Gey KF, Brubacher GB, Stdhelin HB (1987). Plasma levels of antioxidant vitamins in relation to ischaemic heart disease and cancer. *Amer J Clin Nutr* **45 (Suppl 5):** 1368–77.

Eichholzer-Helbling M, Stahelin HB (1991). Plasma antioxidant vitamins and cancer risk: 12-year follow up of the Basle Prospective Study. *Int J Vit Nutr Res* **61:** 271.

West CE and Van Staveren WA (1988). ECP-EURONUT intestinal metaplasia study: Design of the study with special reference to the development and validation of the questionnaire. In *Gastric Carcinogenesis* (eds Reed PI, Hill MJ); Excerpta Medica, Amsterdam pp 229–34.

Reed PI (1990). N-nitroso compounds, gastric carcinogenesis and chemoprevention. In *New Trends in Gastric Cancer: Background and Videosurgery* (eds Reed PI, Carboni M, Johnston BJ, Guadagni S); Kluwer Academic Publishers, Dordrecht/Boston/London, pp 21–30.

UK Subgroup, ECP-EURONUT-IM Study Group (1991). Serum selenium concentrations in patients with intestinal metaplasia and in controls. *Eur J Canc Preven* **1:** 31–4.

Reed PI, Johnston BJ, Walters CL, Hill MJ (1989). Effect of ascorbic acid on the intragastric environment in patients at increased risk of developing gastric cancer. *Gastroenterology* **96:** A411.

Krytopoulos S (1984). Nitrosamines in the environment. Health dangers and intervention possibilities. In *Environmental Carcinogens. The problem in Greece*. Proc Panhellenic Congress of Greek Society of Preventive Medicine, March 1984.

Correa P (1991). Is gastric carcinoma an infectious disease? *New Engl J Med* **325:** 1170–71.

Forman D (1991). The etiology of gastric cancer. In *Relevance to human cancer of N-nitroso compounds, tobacco smoke and mycotoxins* (eds O'Neill IK, Chen J, Bartsch H); Scient Publ No 105, IARC, Lyon, pp 22–32.

Parsonnet J, Friedman GD, Vandersteen DP, Chang Y, Vogelman JH, Orentreich N, Sibley RK (1991). Helicobacter pylori infection and the risk of gastric carcinoma. *New Engl J Med* **325:** 1127–31.

Nomura A, Stemmermann GN, Chyon P-H, Kato I, Perez-Perez GI, Blazer MJ (1991). *Helicobacter pylori* infection and gastric carcinoma among Japanese Americans in Hawaii. *New Engl J Med* **325:** 1132–6

CHAPTER 9

Fibre and Resistant Starch and Cancer

AR LEEDS

Department of Nutrition, King's College London, London W8, UK

'Dietary Fibre' was defined in the 1970's as 'plant polysaccharides' and lignin not digested by enzymes in the small intestine of man (Trowell *et al.*, 1976). This 'physiological' definition is unsatisfactory for a number of reasons, and the development of several different (chemical) analytical methods for dietary fibre has drawn attention to the need for newer chemically specific terms (Marlett, 1990). 'Non-Starch Polysaccharides' is the term currently adopted in the United Kingdom, following the recommendation by a British Nutrition Foundation Taskforce that the term 'Dietary Fibre' be no longer used, at least by the scientific community (British Nutrition Foundation, 1990).

Thus a new classification of plant polysaccharides has been developed, based on chemical composition and also digestibility. This new 'nutritional' classification of plant polysaccharides may help to account for the lack of consistency of the evidence linking colon cancer rates and dietary fibre in the diet. Plant polysaccharides are divided into two main groups: starch – the major carbohydrate of dietary grains and other staple foods – is susceptible to hydrolysis by pancreatic α-amylase, while non-starch polysaccharide (NSP) completely resists digestion by the enzymes of the small intestine of man. It has always been assumed that starch is completely digested and that NSP is completely undigested, however recent evidence indicates that neither of these assumptions is true. Some starch passes into the colon where it may become substrate for colonic fermentation (Bingham, 1990) and some NSP is degraded in the small intestine in some animals.

Studies in man, using an ileostomy model (Englyst and Cummings, 1985, 1986, 1987) have shown that when standardized amounts of starchy foods were fed as single meals to patients whose small gut drained via an ileostomy bag, undigested starch passed out of the small gut. A patient with an ileostomy is not necessarily a good model for intact man, but there was no reason to think that intestinal motility or the level of bacterial colonization were abnormal in the cases used. The NSP recovery matched the amounts of NSP fed almost perfectly, whereas contrary to expectation some starch was recovered, especially after consumption of bananas and cooled potatoes. The term resistant starch was developed during investigation of abnormally high levels of 'NSP' found in breads and potatoes after cooking (Englyst and Cummings, 1985, 1987). The levels were higher in the cooked foods than in the raw foods – clearly an artifact of some kind. Investigation revealed that the excess 'NSP' was composed of glucose and it was concluded that the technique for measuring NSP was at that stage including as NSP a fraction of the starch which was not extracted by the preliminary digestion procedures. The term 'resistant starch' was applied to this fraction.

Subsequent investigation has resulted in a classification of resistant starch into three sub-fractions (Englyst and Kingman, 1990). Physically inaccessible starch occurs within undisrupted plant structures, for example whole or partly milled grains and seeds. The cellular structure may prevent swelling and dispersion of the starch, thus preventing hydrolysis. It is known that coarsely milled grains and food products made from them result in smaller blood glucose and insulin responses suggesting that digestive processing of the starch is slowed and possibly incomplete. After meals of coarsely milled grains a high percentage of faecal solids may be starch which has passed undigested through the gut. Starch occurs in plants in granular structures, and the starch within the granule is in one of three crystalline forms. The type of crystalline structure determines the ease with which amylase gains access to the molecule and achieves hydrolysis. The granule is of course disrupted by cooking so that the amount of 'resistant' starch present in a raw food is not relevant to the question of digestibility if that food is usually eaten cooked. However, if, as is the case with bananas, the food is usually eaten raw, then the presence of resistant starch granules is very important. The crystalline structure of starch is temperature dependent. Gelatinized starch on cooling may form one of the crystalline structures (the B type) which is relatively resistant to hydrolysis by amylase. Thus cooked potatoes, subsequently cooled and eaten without reheating may contain quite a high percentage of starch which cannot be digested in the small gut and which then becomes substrate for fermentation in the colon. This type of resistant starch is termed retrograded starch (Table 1). With regard to the fraction of starch it is clear that the rates of breakdown vary and an arbitrary division into rapidly digestible and slowly digestible starch has been made. This division is based on the amount of glucose released (in the test tube) by digestion of starch with amylase in 20 minutes (rapidly digestible starch) and the amount released between 20 and 120 minutes (slowly digestible starch) (Englyst and Kingman, 1990).

Table 1 Nutritional classification of starch

Rapidly digestible starch (RDS)
Slowly (but completely) digestible starch (SDS)
Resistant starch (RS)
  Physically inaccessible starch (RS1)
  Resistant starch granules (RS2)
  Retrograded starch (RS3)

How is this discussion of starch digestibility relevant to colon cancer? In the absence of extensive analytical data on starch types in many different foods, by methods of analysis which have been thoroughly established and fully validated most of the discussion must be speculative. Data on types of starch present in foods is being generated – in a few years time several sets of data on the composition of commonly consumed starchy foods will be available. An international comparative study on the methods is now underway.

The basis for previous investigations of a possible role for 'dietary fibre' in colon cancer has been the idea that the fibre became a substrate for bacterial fermentation in the colon, increasing stool bulk and shortening transit time. It has been disappointing that the many extensive epidemiological studies have not given consistent results (Faivre, 1992). But perhaps 'dietary fibre' was not the correct measure with which to compare the tumour rates. If resistant starch contributed substrate for fermentation and if fermentation of resistant starch tended to give more butyrate (which is a preferred energy substrate for the lower gut (Roediger, 1980) and which may have an anti-proliferative effect (Kruh, 1982) than fermentation of NSP, then failing to include resistant starch in the comparisons was the reason for the lack of consistency. Perhaps surveys in the future should measure:

Non-Starch Polysaccharide (NSP) + Resistant Starch (RS)

A figure illustrating NSP and RS compositions of some common foods (Figure 1) shows how there are some foods which have low NSP levels, but high (NSP + RS) levels. Populations taking such foods might be deemed as on a relatively low fibre diet, but in fact may well be supplying plenty of substrate to their colons. By contrast some foods containing little resistant starch, but reasonable levels of NSP, may not be such good suppliers of substrate to the colon as might be thought from their NSP content.

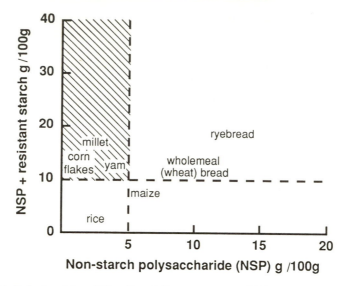

Figure 1 Relationship of Non-Starch Polysaccharide (NSP) content and NSP plus Resistant Starch content of some common foods. The hatched area is the zone in which foods which are relatively low in total NSP but high in NSP plus Resistant Starch are located

How are these Ideas about Starch Digestibility to be Applied to Prevention of Colon Cancer?

In the United Kingdom a new set of dietary reference values (recommended dietary amounts) has been published (Department of Health, 1991). For the first time a recommendation for NSP has been made. The scientific basis for the figures given for NSP was the relationship between stool weights and colon cancer incidence, and between stool weights and colon motility (and the incidence of complaints about constipation) (Table 2). The relationship between dietary fibre-pentose intake and colon cancer rates was also considered and the relationship between NSP intakes and stool weights. Taking account of the present intakes in the UK (11–13 g/d using the Englyst method of analysis) it was calculated that a 50% increase in NSP intake (to about 18 g/d) would increase stool weight by about 25%. This was expected to reduce the proportion of the population with stool weights below 100 g/d who were thus at high risk of colon cancer. It was not the purpose of the report to translate the scientific recommendation into practical advice, but clearly to achieve a 50% increase in NSP requires quite a radical change in the pattern of consumption of cereal products, fruit and vegetables in the United Kingdom. Quite properly at the time of

Table 2 Basis for UK dietary reference value for NSP

Stool weights below 150 g/d associated with colon cancer

Stool weights below 100 g/d associated with complaints
of constipation

(46% UK population pass <100 g/d stool)

NSP intakes of <12 g/d associated with stool
weights of <100 g/d

Present UK NSP intake: 11–13 g/d
(50% from vegetables, 40% from cereals)

Increasing NSP to 18 g/d ($\sim$50% increase) will increase
average stool weight by $\sim$25% and reduce numbers
with stool wts <100 g/d

their deliberations the committee did not make any recommendation about resistant starch.

To make numerical recommendations about the need for carbohydrate for fermentation requires more information than is presently available. Even data based on starch digestion studies performed in the laboratory may not give clear guidance on what really happens in the kitchens and the bowels of those at risk.

Processing of foods which determines particle size etc; ripeness of fruits determines the state of the starch; storage of starchy foods at different temperatures influences starch digestibility; completeness of cooking and the effects of cooling are critical.

It is clear that precise measurements of all of these variables may never be possible on a sufficiently extensive scale to allow the precise nature of the best possible starchy diet to be defined. However, on the basis of what is known it may be worth considering giving some general advice perhaps along the following lines:

- The objective (in countries like the UK where stool weights are low) is to achieve a shift in the distribution of stool weight and transit time in the population.

- Figures can be given for target levels of NSP needed to achieve the necessary changes.

- Foods containing relatively high amounts of resistant starch could be identified qualitatively rather than quantitatively, e.g. rye breads, some legume seeds, as being especially effective for stool bulking and thus might be strongly recommended.

Clearly the present view on 'dietary fibre' and colon cancer is that the evidence at the present time does not allow a strong statement to be made, but perhaps in a few years time when more is known about the significance of resistant starch in stool bulking, colon transit and other colon functions perhaps strong statements about the preventive role of cereals, fruit and vegetables may be possible.

References

Bingham SA (1990). Starch, nonstarch polysaccharides and the large gut. In *Dietary Fibre: Chemistry, Physiology and Health Effects* (eds Kritchevsky D, Bonfield C, Anderson JW); Plenum Press, New York, pp 447–54.

British Nutrition Foundation (1990). Complex Carbohydrates in Foods, the Report of the British Nutrition Foundation's Task Force; Chapman and Hall, London pp 1–2, 137–8.

Department of Health (UK) (1991). Non-starch polysaccharides. In *Dietary Reference Values for Food Energy and Nutrients for the United Kingdom: Report of the Panel on Dietary Reference Values of the Committee on Medical Aspects of Food Policy*. Her Majesty's Stationery Office, London, pp 61–71.

Englyst HN, Cummings JH (1985). Digestion of the polysaccharides of some cereal foods in the human small intestine. *Am J Clin Nutr* 42: 778–87.

Englyst HN, Cummings JH (1986). Digestion of the carbohydrates of banana (*Musa paradisiaca sapientum*) in the human small intestine. *Am J Clin Nutr* 44: 42–50.

Englyst HN, Cummings JH (1987). Digestion of polysaccharides of potato in the small intestine of man. *Am J Clin Nutr* 45: 423–31.

Englyst HN, Kingman S (1990). Dietary Fibre and Resistant Starch: a nutritional classification of plant polysaccharides. In *Dietary Fiber: Chemistry, Physiology and Health Effects* (eds Kritchevsky D, Bonfield C, Anderson JW); Plenum Press, New York, pp 49–65.

Faivre J (1992). Diet and colorectal cancer. See this volume.

Kruh J (1982). Effects of sodium butyrate, a new pharmacological agent, on cells in culture. *Mol Cell Biochem* 42: 65–82.

Marlett JA (1990). Analysis of dietary fiber in human foods. In *Dietary Fiber: Chemistry, Physiology and Health Effects* (eds Kritchevsky D, Bonfield C, Anderson JW); Plenum Press, New York, pp 31–48.

Roediger WEW (1980). Role of anaerobic bacteria in the metabolic welfare of the colonic mucosa in man. *Gut* 21: 793–8.

Trowell H *et al*. (1976). Dietary fibre redefined. *Lancet* 1: 967.

CHAPTER 10

Public Education on Diet and Cancer: Calories, Weight and Exercise

C LA VECCHIA[1,2], E NEGRI[1]

[1] *Istituto di Ricerche Farmacologiche "Mario Negri",*
Via Eritrea 62, 20157 Milano, Italy
[2] *Institute of Social and Preventive Medicine, University of Lausanne,*
1005 Lausanne, Switzerland *

Introduction

The observation that energy intake, and consequently body weight, have a role in the process of carcinogenesis was made in the early 1940's on animal experiments: rodents fed *at libitum* had a higher cancer incidence than animals with restricted calorie intake (Tannenbaum, 1940).

It is much simpler to analyse energy balance in animals, however, than in the complexity of human life, and the application of these observations to human cancer incidence is therefore not obvious. In particular, both interpretations – that overfeeding is associated with increased cancer risk, or that calorie restriction is related to decreased risk – seemed plausible.

This review will therefore be restricted to human evidence, and discuss available data and open questions on calories, weight, height, exercise and cancer risk, with specific attention to prevention and public health education.

Calories

Calorie intake is one of the most difficult issues to quantify and investigate, since extensive and detailed questionnaires are required to obtain a reliable measure of total energy intake. Further, validation of data collec-

* Correspondence should be addressed to: C La Vecchia MD, Istituto di Ricerche Farmacologiche "Mario Negri", Via Eritrea, 62–20157 Milan, Italy. Tel: 02–390141; Fax: 02–3546277

tion is complex and difficult, too, since a large number of different foods are involved (Willett *et al.*, 1985a; 1986; Pietinen *et al.*, 1988a; 1988b).

However, allowance for total calories is an important methodological point for any analysis and inference on the independent role of other nutrients (fats, proteins, etc.) or micronutrients (vitamins, minerals, etc). For the purpose of using calories as a covariate, however, Willett and Stampfer (1986) postulated that even an approximate measure may be useful, and simply defined calories as the sum of carbohydrates, fats, proteins plus alcohol. Such approximation for the purpose of estimating disease risk is meant more to rank subjects correctly as concerns their caloric intake than to provide absolute measurement of daily calories.

Although the uncertainties regarding total energy measures are substantial, there is some indication that elevated intake can be related to cancer risk in humans. Different studies observed an association for breast cancer, and there are some data for colorectal cancer, too (Willett, 1989; Potter and McMichael, 1986).

Since total calories are the sum of three main components (carbohydrates, fats and proteins), not surprisingly most studies tended to observe stronger associations for one or another of these components, and most often with the main one, fats (and probably aetiologically the most important one).

Epidemiological data are therefore still open to debate, and probably will remain so in the near future, particularly since two major prospective studies found no association between energy, fats and breast cancer risk (Willett *et al.*, 1987; Jones *et al*, 1987). Thus, although these indications find some plausible support in experimental data on rodents, the overall evidence on calorie intake *per se* and human cancer risk is too scant to allow definition and implementation of public education interventions, in the absence of excess weight.

Weight

There is substantial evidence that overweight and obesity are related to at least three cancer sites: gallbladder, endometrium and breast in post-menopausal women (Lew and Garfinkel, 1979). The relative risks are of the order of five for obese individuals as compared to leaner ones for gallbladder and endometrium, but only about 30–50% higher for breast cancer (Table 1). Still, since mortality rates from breast cancer are substantially higher than from gallbladder and endometrial neoplasms, the public health implications of elevated breast cancer rates in overweight individuals are probably greater than for any other neoplasms.

The underlying aetiological mechanisms are different for gallbladder as compared to breast or endometrial cancer. Obesity, in fact, is a major cause

Table 1 **Mortality ratios for selected sites of cancer. The American Cancer Society One Million Study (Lew *et al.*, 1979)**

Site	<80	80–89	90–109	110–119	120–129	130–139	≥140
			Weight Index				
MALES							
Stomach	134	61	100	122	97	73	188
Colorectum	90	86	100	126	123	153	173
Pancreas	120	82	100	91	88	76	162
Kidney	106	96	100	163	139	191	—
Prostate	102	92	100	90	137	133	129
FEMALES							
Stomach	74	95	100	107	126	126	103
Colorectum	93	84	100	96	110	130	122
Breast	82	86	100	119	116	122	153
Cervix	76	77	100	124	151	142	239
Endometrium	89	109	100	136	185	230	542
Ovary	86	98	100	115	99	88	163
Kidney	112	70	100	109	130	185	203

of gallstones (La Vecchia, 1991a), and this is likely to be the basis of the elevated risk of gallbladder cancer, too, while for cancers of the breast and mostly of the endometrium, the underlying biological mechanisms are related to the increased oestrogen levels in post-menopausal obese women, due to aromatization of androgens to oestrogens in the adipose tissue (La Vecchia *et al.*, 1988).

A hormonal mechanism, although still largely undefined, is probably at the basis of the possible association between overweight and cancer of the prostate, which is of similar magnitude (and public health importance) to that with breast cancer, although published evidence is not totally consistent (Table 2) (La Vecchia *et al.*, 1991a; 1988).

Further, the American Cancer Society One Million Cohort Study (Lew and Garfinkel, 1979), the cohort of 50,000 American Alumni (Whittemore *et al.*, 1985) and some (Goodman *et al.*, 1986) though not all (Talamini *et al.*, 1991) case-control studies found a direct association between measures of body weight and renal cell adenocarcinoma. Besides epidemiological confirmation, this possible association lacks clear understanding of potential biological mechanism(s), but would be of interest, particularly since little is known on the causes of adenocarcinoma of the kidney, besides an association with smoking (La Vecchia *et al.*, 1991b).

94 Public Education on Diet and Cancer

Table 2 Relation of body mass index with cancer of the breast, endometrium and prostate from a series of case-control studies conducted in Northern Italy (La Vecchia *et al.*, 1988)

| Body mass index (kg/m²) | Relative risk (95% confidence interval) for: | | |
	Breast cancer	Endometrial cancer	Prostatic cancer
<20	1*	1*	1*
20–24	1.3 (0.9–1.0)	1.6 (1.0–2.5)	
25–29	1.2 (0.9–1.7)	2.4 (1.5–3.8)	2.0 (1.2–3.5)
≥30	1.6 (1.1–2.4)	6.4 (3.9–10.4)	2.5 (1.2–5.2)

*Reference category

It is more difficult, particularly using a case-control approach, to study the relationship between measures of body weight and digestive tract sites, since early symptoms of these neoplasms induce modifications of dietary patterns and hence body weight changes (La Vecchia, 1990). It is thus conceivable, though not proven, that overweight may have some influence on colorectal cancer too, as well as on other tumours linked to neoplastic cachexia, such as pancreas and ovary. All these sites, in fact, were linked to overweight in the American Cancer Society One Million Cohort Study (Lew and Garfinkel, 1979) (Table 1).

These uncertainties and the limitations of published work still cannot eclipse the importance, on a public health scale, of overweight and obesity as a cause of human cancer. In the United States, in fact, it has been estimated that approximately 2% of all cancer deaths are due to overweight (Doll and Peto, 1981). Although in Europe this proportion may be somewhat lower, this is not only relevant from a public health viewpoint, but also has important and immediate implications for prevention. Overweight is the single aspect of nutrition and diet to be so well-defined in epidemiological terms as to open immediate perspectives for intervention and prevention, and on which public education could have useful effects.

Besides cancer, moreover, education and campaigns against overweight and obesity also have major consequences for other major groups of diseases, from diabetes to cardiovascular to digestive tract conditions (Garfinkel *et al.*, 1988).

Height

Adult height, although largely genetically determined, is influenced by nutrition early in life too. Thus, as an indicator, however indirect, of nutritional status in childhood and adolescence, it is relevant for its potential correlates with adult cancer risk.

In the early 1970's a Dutch prospective study (De Waard and Baanders-van Halewijn, 1974) showed an association between stature and post-menopausal breast cancer that was independent of weight: the relative risk rose to 3.6 for tallest/heaviest women compared to the lowest height/weight category. Subsequent studies of height and breast cancer (Swanson et al., 1988; Warren, 1980; Willett et al., 1985b; Parazzini et al., 1990) produced inconsistent results but, at least from an aetiological viewpoint, it is important that height and weight are considered separately as well as in terms of combined indexes (De Waard and Trichopoulos, 1988; La Vecchia, 1989).

In the cohort study of the First National Health and Nutrition Examination Survey (NHANES 1) (Albanes et al., 1988) elevated rates were observed for breast cancer in females and intestinal cancer and all sites in males. Further, a prospective study from Hawaii suggested that measures of body height might be related to the incidence of prostatic cancer (Severson et al., 1988) and two case-control studies from the United States (Winder et al., 1966) and Greece (Koumantaki et al., 1989) found an association between stature and the risk of endometrial cancer.

The relationship between height and cancer risk was examined systematically within the framework of a case-control surveillance of several cancer sites conducted in Northern Italy (La Vecchia et al., 1990). No significant direct association emerged, and there was only a suggestion of elevated prostatic cancer risk in males in the highest quintile of height. In contrast a few inverse associations were observed, with oesophageal, cervical and endometrial cancer, suggesting that a poorer diet early in life may be an unfavourable indicator of subsequent risk for a few cancer sites too (Table 3).

Some of the inconsistencies between various studies may be due to the different importance of nutrition in childhood and adolescence for adult height in various populations, particularly with reference to different levels of dietary deficiencies in the past (La Vecchia et al., 1990). Other inconsistencies are more difficult to explain, and probably at least in part attributable to the varying aspect of chance or bias on a relatively mild association.

The issue of height and cancer risk has clear relevance from an aetio-pathogenic viewpoint, and potential implications for intervention and cancer prevention for future generations, although, even if the potential

**Table 3 Relative risk of selected cancer sites according to height Milan, Italy 1983–89
(La Vecchia *et al.*, 1990)**

Type of cancer	Sex	Relative risk estimates for height quintile				
		1* *(Lowest)*	*2*	*3*	*4*	*5* *(Highest)*
Oesophagus	M	1	0.9	0.5	0.6	0.7*
Stomach	M	1	1.3	1.0	1.3	1.0
Colon	M	1	1.1	1.0	1.3	1.3
	F	1	1.1	0.9	0.8	0.8
Rectum	M	1	1.0	0.9	1.1	1.2
	F	1	2.1	1.0	1.4	0.8
Breast	F	1	1.1	1.0	1.1	1.0
Cervix	F	1	0.7	0.6	0.5	0.4*
Endometrium	F	1	0.9	0.9	0.7	0.7*
Prostate	M	1	1.1	1.3	1.5	1.6

*$p<0.05$

association between height and the risk of some cancer site is confirmed, any measure of reduction of stature for cancer prevention is unlikely to be proposed and socially accepted.

Physical exercise

This is the less directly and extensively studied aspect of energy balance, and only scattered indications are available. Epidemiologically, there are major difficulties in studying exercise. Occupational exercise, in fact, is strongly correlated to social class and hence to a wide range of other environmental and lifestyle exposures. Leisure time exercise is also confounded, though to a lesser extent, by social class indicators, and can be a consequence, as well as a cause, of general health conditions.

To further complicate the issue, physical activity is difficult to study and quantify and the related methods of analysis have not received major attention by epidemiologists.

Consequently, most published work relies on proxy indicators of physical exercise, such as occupation or number of children, assuming for instance that young children represent a considerable burden in terms of physical activity. Using such indirect measures, a few studies have tended to suggest an inverse association between physical activity and colorectal cancer risk (Willett, 1989; Garfinkel and Stellman, 1988; Ballard-Barbash *et al.*, 1990; Whittemore *et al.*, 1990; Albanes *et al.*, 1989). This may well find some biological interpretation in terms of fast faecal transit in the large bowel with higher physical activity, but it remains, at present, a useful and interesting hypothesis more than an established association; particularly since the relationship was moderate and inconsistent in other studies (Whittemore *et al.*, 1990; Albanes *et al.*, 1989). Likewise, the reduced breast cancer risk among ballet dancers or other groups of women with high physical activity in adolescence has been generally interpreted in terms of the effect of body mass (and related hormonal factors), on breast carcinogenesis, rather than of direct relation to physical activity (Frisch *et al.*, 1987).

To complicate any inference, some of the direct epidemiological observations are inconsistent with the hypothesis that physical exercise reduces cancer incidence. The American Cancer Society One Million Cohort Study (Garfinkel and Stellman, 1988) for instance, found reduced standardized mortality ratios (SMR) for all causes and ischaemic heart disease in subjects reporting heavy exercise, but elevated cancer rates in women (SMR = 120) for all causes, and for cancers of the lung, colorectum and pancreas in both sexes (Table 4). Likewise, in a cohort study of over 50,000 alumni, physical activity ($\geq$5 hours per week) was associated with reduced rectal cancer risk (relative risk, RR=0.6, 95% confidence interval, 90.2–1.0), but with elevated prostatic cancer risk (RR=1.7, 95% Cl 1.1–2.6) (Whittemore *et al.*, 1985). Again, confounding cannot be excluded, but these data clearly do not support the view that heavy physical exercise *per se* reduces cancer risk. In the NHANES 1 cohort study (Albanes *et al*, 1989), the risk of all cancers, colorectal and lung cancer was elevated among inactive males, when non-recreational activity was considered, but the pattern was different for recreational activity and in females, indicating the possibility of confounding by social class.

Table 4 Standardized mortality ratios (SMR) for selected causes for subjects reporting heavy exercise. Data from the American Cancer Society One Million Study (Garfinkel and Stellman, 1988)

Cause of death	Males	Females
All causes	92	94
Ischaemic heart disease	88	64
Cerebrovascular disease	80	87
All cancers	99	120
Lung cancer	119	136
Colorectal cancer	122	137
Pancreatic cancer	122	137

Consequently, major methodological issues have to be tackled before establishing and quantifying the potential impact of physical activity *per se* (i.e. independent from obesity and energy balance) on human cancer risk and hence before defining indications for prevention and public education.

Conclusions

The factors considered in this presentation are closely related, and this alone would by itself complicate any analysis aimed at disentangling their separate effects on the risk of human cancers. To further complicate the issue, one of these factors (weight) is relatively easy to measure and analyse, although systematic tendencies to under-report weight have been observed, and early symptoms of the disease or other possible sources of misclassification can introduce further errors.

Still, the evidence from case-control and cohort studies associating overweight and obesity with a number of important cancer sites is consistent enough to allow reliable estimates of relative risks and reasonable estimates of population attributable risks. Thus, public education to reduce overweight and obesity is not only possible, but should clearly be considered a public health priority.

Epidemiological data are much more scattered and confused for height, which has been taken as an indirect indicator of nutrition in childhood and adolescence, and the other two points of the picture, calories and exercise. It is possible that some of this confusion is due to the difficulty in measuring these variables, and that some of these issues may be clarified and quantified in the future. At present, however, there is only some indication that high calorie intake may be associated with breast and colorectal cancer risk, while higher physical activity may protect against large intestinal cancer.

In developed countries, reduced caloric intake and greater physical activity may be beneficial for other important groups of diseases, including cardiovascular diseases, metabolic and gastro-intestinal conditions (Garfinkel and Stellman, 1988). On these grounds alone, therefore, one could argue that public education campaigns are justified. This is, however, a matter of health policy rather than of scientific debate, and its potential advantages should be weighed against its possible drawbacks, since the number of public education strategies against cancer in our society has to be limited, and priorities have to be given. Overweight and obesity are certainly among these priorities.

Acknowledgements

This work was conducted within the framework of the National Research Council (CNR), Applied Projects "Oncology" (Contract No 870154444) and "Risk Factors for Disease" and with the contribution of the Italian Association for Cancer Research and the Italian League against tumours, Milan. The Authors wish to thank Mrs J Baggott, Mrs MP Bonifacino and the GA Pfeiffer Memorial Library for editorial assistance.

References

Albanes D, Jones DY, Schatzkin A, Micozzi MS, Taylor PR (1988). Adult stature and risk of cancer. *Cancer Res* **48**: 1658–62.

Albanes D, Balir A, Taylor PR (1989). Physical activity and risk of cancer in the NHANES 1 population. *Am J Public Health* **79**: 744–50.

Ballard-Barbash R, Schatzkin A, Albanes D *et al*. (1990). Physical activity and risk of large bowel cancer in the Framingham Study. *Cancer Res* **50**: 3610–3.

De Waard F, Baanders-van Halewijn EA (1974). A prospective study in general practice on breast cancer risk in postmenopausal women. *Int J Cancer* **14**: 153–60.

De Waard F, Trichopoulos D (1988). A unifying concept of the aetiology of breast cancer. *Int J Cancer* **41**: 666–9.

Doll R, Peto R (1981). The causes of cancer: Quantitative estimates of avoidable risks of cancer in United States today. *J Natl Cancer Inst* **66**: 1191–308.

Frisch RE, Wyshak G, Albright NL *et al*. (1987). Lower lifetime occurrence of breast cancer and cancers of the reproductive system among former college athletes. *Am J Clin Nutr* **45**: 328–35.

Garfinkel L, Stellman SD (1988). Mortality by relative weight and exercise. *Cancer* **62**: 1844–50.

Goodman MT, Morgenstern H, Wynder EL (1986). A case-control study of factors affecting the development of renal cell cancer. *Am J Epidemiol* **124**: 926–41.

Jones DY, Schatzkin A, Green SB *et al*. (1987). Dietary fat and breast cancer in the National Health and Nutrition Examination Survey I Epidemiologic Follow-up Study. *JNCI* **89**: 465–71.

Koumantaki Y, Tzonou A, Koumantakis E, Kaklamani E, Aravantinos D, Trichopoulos D (1989). A case-control study of cancer of endometrium in Athens. *Int J Cancer* **43**: 795–9.

La Vecchia C, Decarli A, Negri E, Parazzini F (1988). Epidemiological aspects of diet and cancer: A summary review of case-control studies from Northern Italy. *Oncology* **45**: 364–70.

La Vecchia C (1989). Nutritional factors and cancers of the breast, endometrium and ovary. *Eur J Cancer Clin Oncol* **25**: 1945-51.

La Vecchia C, Negri E, Parazzini F *et al*. (1990). Height and cancer risk in a network of case-control studies from Northern Italy. *Int J Cancer* **45**: 275–9.

La Vecchia C, Negri E, D'Avanzo B, Boyle P (1991a). Risk factors for gallstone disease requiring surgery. *Int J Epidemiol*.

La Vecchia C, Negri E, D'Avanzo B, Franceschi S (1991b). Smoking and renal cell carcinoma. *Cancer Res*.

Lew EA, Garfinkel L (1979). Variations in mortality by weight among 750,000 men and women. *J Chronic Dis* 32: 563–76.

Parazzini F, La Vecchia C, Negri E, Bruzzi P, Palli D, Boyle P (1990). Anthropometric variables and risk of breast cancer. *Int J Cancer* 45: 397–402.

Pietinen P, Hartman AM, Haapa E *et al.* (1988a). Reproducibility and validity of dietary assessment instruments. I. A self-administered food use questionnaire with a portion size picture booklet. *Am J Epidemiol* 128: 655–66.

Pietinen P, Hartman AM, Haapa E *et al.* (1988b). Reproducibility and validity of dietary assessment instruments. II. A qualitative food frequency questionnaire. *Am J Epidemiol* 128: 667–76.

Potter JD, McMichael AJ (1986). Diet and cancer of the colon and rectum: A case-control study. *J Natl Cancer Inst* 76: 557–69.

Severson RK, Grove JS, Nomura AMY, Stemmermann GN (1988). Body mass and prostatic cancer: A prospective study. *Br Med J* 297: 713–5.

Swanson CA, Jones DY, Schatzkin A, Brinton LA, Ziegler RG (1988). Breast cancer risk assessed by anthropometry in the NHANES 1 epidemiological follow-up study. *Cancer Res* 48: 5363–7.

Talamini R, Baron AE, Bara S *et al.* (1991). A case-control study of risk factors for renal cell cancer in Northern Italy. *Cancer Causes Control*.

Tannenbaum A (1940). Relationship of body weight to cancer incidence. *Arch Pathol* 30: 509–17.

Warren MP (1980). The effects of exercise on pubertal progression and reproduction on girls. *J Clin Endocrinol Metab* 51: 1150–7.

Whittemore AS, Paffenbarger RS Jr, Anderson K, Lee JE (1985). Early precursors of site-specific cancers in college men and women. *JNCI* 74: 43–51.

Whittemore AS, Wu-Williams AH, Lee M *et al.* (1990). Diet, physical activity and colorectal cancer among Chinese in North America and China. *J Natl Cancer Inst* 82: 915–26.

Willett WC, Sampson L, Stampfer MJ *et al.* (1985a). Reproducibility and validity of a semiquantitative food frequency questionnaire. *Am J Epidemiol* 122: 51–65.

Willett WC, Browne ML, Bain C *et al.* (1985b). Relative weight and risk of breast cancer among premenopausal women. *Am J Epidemiol* 122: 731–40.

Willett W, Stampfer MJ (1986). Total energy intake: Implications for epidemiologic analyses. *Am J Epidemiol* 124: 17–27.

Willett WC, Stampfer MJ, Colditz GA *et al.* (1987). Dietary fat and the risk of breast cancer. *N Engl J Med* 316: 22–8.

Willett W (1989). The search for the causes of breast and colon cancer. *Nature* 338: 389–94.

Winder E, Escher G, Mantel N (1966). An epidemiologic investigation of cancer of the endometrium. *Cancer* 19: 489–520.

CHAPTER 11

Dietary Fats and Cancer – an Update

PA JUDD

Department of Nutrition and Dietetics
King's College, London, UK

Introduction

The term dietary fat covers a wide range of materials found in foods. In the past fat in the diet was important mainly because the major triglyceride component supplied a concentrated form of energy and because the fat also often carried many of the volatile flavouring compounds in food, thereby providing this energy in a palatable form. However, fat is not simply an energy supply – it has become apparent, firstly through the research into the role of different fatty acids in heart disease and increasingly in other health areas that different groups of fatty acids may have different physiological effects. Thus fatty acids with different chain lengths and degrees of saturation may be metabolized in subtly different ways which may be of benefit or otherwise to health. Recently the fact that different series of fatty acids (i.e. the $\omega 3$ and $\omega 6$ fatty acids) are metabolized in particular ways has also been seen as important.

Fats in foods are also intimately bound with other substances such as cholesterol and the fat soluble vitamins A, D, E and K and as research continues it has become obvious that the relationships between these nutrients are complex even before the possible modulating effects of associated intake of other dietary components such as complex carbohydrates and non-starch polysaccharides are considered.

Exploration of the relationship between fats in the diet and a group of diseases such as cancers is therefore more complicated when all the above factors are to be taken into consideration. Measuring the total fat intake in most diets is notoriously difficult. It has been estimated that between 7 and 10 days of dietary records are required to reliably classify individuals into extreme tertiles of fat intake and up to 23 days for cholesterol (Marr and Heady, 1986). Studies comparing fat intakes calculated from food tables and comparing these with analysis of duplicate diets demonstrate how difficult it is to obtain accurate information especially when attempts are made to identify the different types of fatty acids. Similar problems arise with estimation of other nutrients such as the fat soluble vitamins and cholesterol. In epidemiological studies dietary data are collected at a much less sensitive level than in individual studies and data should always be interpreted with careful consideration of the methodology used. A detailed consideration of the methodological issues in studying the relationship between dietary fat and cancer has been presented by Mettlin (1986).

Despite the problems a large amount of data has been collected regarding the likelihood of associations between dietary fat intake and various cancers. Epidemiological methods used include comparing populations through inter-country correlation studies where per capita fat consumption is compared with cancer in incidence; case control studies for particular cancers; prospective cohort studies and intervention trials. In 1985 at the conclusion of an ECP symposium on diet and cancer the evidence for the role of dietary fat in the aetiology of several cancers was considered firm enough to make the following statement with respect to fat:

> Decrease the intake of saturated and unsaturated fat in countries where on average fat constitutes more than 30% of total food energy (calories). In other countries, people should maintain their lower fat intake.

The present paper will examine evidence which has emerged since this consensus statement appeared mainly with respect to those cancers said to be hormone-related such as breast, ovarian, endometrial and prostate cancer and colorectal cancer, for which logical hypotheses for the role of fat in the aetiology have been expressed.

Dietary Fat and Endocrine-Associated Cancers

The role of dietary fats in the aetiology of the group including cancer of the breast, endometrium, ovary and prostate is perhaps more complex and controversial than it appeared a few years ago. Although the observation that differences in cancer incidence and mortality exist in different parts of the world or within countries (Muir *et al.*, 1987) and the possible associations with diet have apparently been well accepted (Armstrong and Doll, 1975) it has recently been suggested that many studies which found associations between diet and endocrine – related cancers were flawed methodologically. Berrino *et al.* (1989) reviewed the epidemiological studies relating dietary factors to cancer of hormone dependent organs, examining the data published to that date in terms of the reliability or validity of the data and concluded that only one third of the studies could be regarded as reliable.

Breast Cancer

When between-country comparisons are made mortality from breast cancer shows a strong correlation with per capita intake of total fat (Armstrong and Doll, 1975; Goodwin and Boyd, 1987). Evidence collected so far suggests that the between and within country differences hold only for the postmenopausal form of the disease, there being little difference in the incidence for women younger than 40 years (De Waard, 1979). Hill (1987) suggests that dietary fat intake is only associated with the postmenopausal form of the disease although there are studies which have shown weak associations in pre-menopausal women. It would seem that related anthropometric measures such as height, weight and Body Mass Intake (BMI) are also most often positively associated with breast cancer incidence in the postmenopausal state (Berrino *et al*, 1989).

However, the results from analytical observational studies designed to test the aetiological hypothesis linking fat and breast cancer could best be described as inconclusive. Berrino lists 21 studies on diet and breast cancer reported between 1975 and 1987. Of these, six studies showed an association between dietary fat intake and breast cancer (see Table 1), and four of these were considered by the reviewers to be reliable studies. Three other studies listed, including the large cohort study of nurses in the USA (Willet *et al.*, 1987), considered the most reliable, showed no association with intake of fat.

One theory suggested to explain the continuing inconsistent results with respect to associations between total fat and breast cancer (Carroll *et al.*, 1986; Wynder *et al.*, 1986; Potter, 1987) is that different types of fats may have different and even opposite effects; a theory which has to some extent been borne out by animal studies (Carroll, 1985). However, few epidemiological studies have employed dietary assessment methods which allow estimation of total calories, total fat and different types of fatty acids. Where this has been the case results are again contradictory. Mill *et al.* (1978) and Howe (1985) suggest that, in premenopausal women, risk of breast cancer was increased in those with a high intake of saturated fat but this was not confirmed by an Australian study although a slightly decreasing risk was demonstrated in premenopausal women with increasing intakes of polyunsaturated fatty acids (Rohan *et al.*, 1988). In Finland Knekt and co-workers (1990) studied 3,988 women whose diets had been measured 20 years previously. Risk of breast cancer was significantly inversely related to energy intake and non-significantly inversely related to absolute fat intake. However a positive association between energy-adjusted fat intake and occurrence of breast cancer was apparent. An attempt to measure different types of fats was made using newly developed food tables and the relative risk for the highest compared to the lowest

Public Education on Diet and Cancer

tertile of intakes was found to be greatest for monounsaturated fats and cholesterol but lower and similar for saturated and polyunsaturated fats.

Many workers have studied intakes of foods as distinct from attempting to measure nutrient intake and again the results are mixed. In some studies meat intake was significantly associated with the disease but in others this was not observed. Where milk and dairy product intake had been examined most studies in the series described by Berrino found a positive association although the recent Finnish study demonstrated the opposite effect (Knekt *et al.*, 1990). Again however this study illustrates the problems of comparing diets between countries. If, as has been suggested

Table 1 Analytical studies on diet and breast cancer

Year	1st Author	Design	No of cases	Total or saturated fats	Meat	Milk & dairy	Vegetable fats	Fruit or vegetables
1987	Willett	cohort	601	na			na	
1988	Toniolo	case/control	250	+	sp	+	na	na
1978/85	Miller/Howe	case/control	400	+ *			– *	
1985	Hirohata	case/control	212	sp			sn	
1987	Hirohata	case/control	344	sp			na	
1986	Hislop	case/control	861		+ *	+ *		– *
1982	Kinlen	cohort	62		sp			
1988	Mills	cohort	186		na	na		
1986	Lubin F	case/control	818	+ *				sn *
1986/88	Katsouyanni	case/control	120		na	na		–
1982	Graham	case/control	2024	na				– *
1984	Talamini	case/control	368		na	+		
1986	Lé	case/control	1010			+		
1987	Jones	cohort	99	–			sn	
1978	Hirayama	cohort	139		+			
1978	Nomura	cohort	86		+	+		
1981	Lubin	case/control	577		+	+		
1975	Philips	case/control	77		na	sp		
1985	Zemla	case/control	328		sp *			– *
1985	Sarin	case/control	68	+				

+   = Significant (*p* <0.05) positive association
–   = Significant (*p* <0.05) negative association
na = No association
sp = Suggestive of positive association
sn = Suggestive negative association
*   = Association limited to subgroups
From Berrino *et al.*, 1989.

previously (Hill, 1987), it is fat from animal sources (especially meat) which is most important it is interesting to note that the proportions of fat provided by meat, milk products and fats and oils in Finland and the USA are very different (21%, 30%, 34% and 38%, 12%, 40% respectively) and it is likely that similar differences can be seen in the diets of other populations.

Hill (1987) has discussed the proposed mechanisms for the tumour-promoting effects of dietary fat and suggested a model for the development of post-menopausal, oestrogen dependent breast cancers (Hill, 1990). The risk of breast cancer is increased by early menarche and late menopause, both of which he suggests are associated with a high fat/high meat/high energy diet. A high fat diet may also increase oestrogen production and increased breast adiposity and thus increase the concentration of oestrogen receptors (Chan and Cohen, 1975).

A recent suggestion is that there may be a cut-off point for total fat intake such that an effect for fat might be observed only below a certain intake (e.g. 50 g/day) and is therefore undetectable in most studies. Most western populations would fall outside this level, although it may help to explain the results in some studies such as the large Japanese prospective study reported by Hirayama (1985). If this theory is correct then it would support the idea of reducing fat intake to less than 30% of energy intake as suggested by ECP in 1985. However for the majority of women in the UK using current recommendations (COMA, 1991) this would still result in an intake of 70 g fat per day.

Endometrial Cancer

Fat intake is positively associated with endometrial cancer in ecological studies (Armstrong and Doll, 1975: Thomas and Chu, 1986). In individual studies, however, there is little direct evidence for an effect of fat or of any other nutrient. A study of lacto-ovo vegetarians, who have similar fat intakes to omnivores but a lower incidence of endometrial cancer has led to the suggestion that meat-derived diets might be implicated (Phillips, 1975). In addition, a case control study carried out in Italy showed that when subjects were asked to estimate whether their intake of fats and oils was high, medium or low the cases were more likely to have higher intakes (La Vecchia *et al.*, 1986). The main positive associations are with indicators of body weight as reviewed by Berrino *et al.* (1989). Obesity has been associated with endometrial cancer in many epidemiological studies, an effect which is suggested to operate by increasing endogenous or exogenous oestrogen levels (Henderson *et al.*, 1988). Early menarche and late menopause are also associated with higher risk of developing endometrial cancer (McMahon, 1974) and thus fat intake may be indirectly implicated due to its importance as an energy source (Ries, 1973).

Ovarian Cancer

Ovarian cancer shares similar geographical correlations with cancer of the breast and endometrium (Armstrong and Doll, 1975; Thomas and Chu, 1986) but the associations with diet are even less clear. It has been suggested that consumption of dairy products is associated with higher risk of ovarian cancer either through an effect of lactose (Cramer, 1989; Cramer *et al.*, 1989) or because of the high fat content of these foods (Cramer *et al.*, 1984). A recent case-control study examined this theory by looking at consumption of different milks in 303 patients with ovarian cancer and 606 age-matched controls and concluded that consumption of whole milk was the most important risk factor via its fat content (Mettlin and Piver, 1990). Snowden (1983) has also suggested a positive association with fat intake but two other recent case control studies looking at both fat intake and body weight gave contradictory results. Byers and co-workers (1983) showed no association with fat intake and a negative association with body weight whereas Cramer (1984) demonstrated a positive association with both animal fat intake and overweight. The large American Cancer Society prospective study showed that only women weighing more than 140% of ideal weight were more at risk of ovarian cancer (Lew and Garfinkel, 1979).

Other studies have been equally contradictory and Berrino (1989), reviewing these, concluded that there is insufficient evidence to come to any conclusions about diet and ovarian cancer.

Prostatic Cancer

The epidemiology of cancer of the prostate has been recently reviewed by Donn and Muir (1985) and discussed by Hill (1987), Berrino *et al.* (1989) and Jenson *et al.* (1990). The incidence and mortality from the disease correlate with other diseases such as breast cancer and uterine cancer and several inter- and intra-country studies show positive correlations with fat intake (Armstrong and Doll, 1975). Wynder *et al.* (1971) showed that fat intake accounted for around 40% of energy intake in high risk areas compared to 20% in low risk areas.

Jenson lists 10 studies relating diet and prostate cancer in which at least 7 show some association between either total fat consumption or foods of animal origin and rich in fat such as meat, dairy products and milk or eggs and incidence of prostate cancer (see Table 2). However, many of these

Table 2 Summary of epidemiological studies examining dietary fat and prostate cancer

1st Authors	Year	Design	No of cases/ controls	Total fat	Meat	Eggs	Milk and dairy
Rotkin #	1977	case/control			PA	PA	PA
Meikel*	1982	case/control				SA	SA
Schuman#	1982	case/control			NA	PA	SA
Graham	1983	case/control	262/259	SA	SA		
Heshmat	1985	case/control	181/181	PA (1)			
Kaul	1987	case/control	55/55	NA (2)			
Kolonel	1988	case/control	452/899	SA (3)			
Ohno	1988	case/control	100/200	NA			
Hirayama	1979	cohort	63/122261		NA		
Snowdon	1984	cohort	99/6763		PA	PA	PA

SA = Significant Association ($p<0.05$)
PA = Positive Association
NA = No Association
(1) = Among men 30–49 years old
(2) = Men 50 years and older, linoleic acid intake was significantly greater
       among controls than cases ($p<0.04$)
(3) = Among men 70 years older
* = Cited by Snowdon
\# = Cited by National Research Council, 1982
From Jenson, 1990.

studies have again been criticized for the crude methods used to estimate diet or for analysis although Berrino suggests that this may mean that the true magnitude of the association may, in fact, be greater. Two of the 3 studies in which no association with fat was seen were carried out in Japan and it has been suggested that the association may be with high levels of meat intake which are rare in Japan (Berrino, 1989). In another Japanese study (Mishina *et al*, 1985) consumption of western foods (and hence high fat foods?) was found to be a risk factor.

Donn and Muir (1985) have proposed that a high fat diet changes the hormone profile as shown by Hill *et al.* (1979) and Heshmat *et al* (1985) and causes an increased uptake of male hormones by the prostate. Hill has suggested a model for the development of prostate cancer where unidentified factors act on the normal prostate, resulting in latent carcinoma. Increased uptake of male hormones and an altered hormone profile (containing higher levels of testosterone) will then promote the development of cancer (Hill, 1990).

Colorectal Cancer

In western countries the incidence of colon cancer is 10 times that in many Far Eastern and developing countries (Doll and Peto, 1981).

There have been a wealth of epidemiological studies regarding diet and colorectal cancer reviewed recently by Jenson (1985). Two main hypotheses (Willett *et al.*, 1984; Zaridze, 1983) have emerged in recent decades i.e. that diets high in fat, especially from animal sources, increase the risk and that a high intake of dietary fibre decreases it. The hypothesis that dietary fat is involved in the causation of colon cancer again derives from the marked inter-country correlations between per capita consumption of animal fat or meat and disease incidence (Armstrong and Doll, 1975; Rose *et al.*, 1986).

In several recent case-control studies where detailed information about diet sufficient to allow calculation of total fat intake has been collected, the majority have found significant positive correlations (Bristol *et al.*, 1985; Potter *et al.*, 1986; Lyon *et al*, 1987; Graham *et al.*, 1988; Kune *et al.*, 1987; Slattery *et al.*, 1988; Whitemore *et al.*, 1990) although three others have not (Berta *et al.*, 1985; Macquart-Moulin, 1986; Tuyns *et al.*, 1987). In several of these studies there have been positive correlations between energy intake and the risk of colon cancer (Jain *et al.*, 1980; Bristol *et al.*, 1985; Potter *et al.*, 1986; Willet and Stampfer, 1986; Lyon *et al.*, 1987; Graham *et al.*, 1988; Slattery *et al.*, 1988). So, as with the hormone dependent cancers it is difficult to come to a conclusion as to whether total food intake or the fat content of the diet is the important factor.

Other authors have suggested that the correlation with fat intake is secondary to the stronger correlation with meat (Haenszel *et al*, 1973) and this would seem to be supported by the calculations done by Draser and Irving in 1973, where 'bound fat', mainly from meat, appears to account for many of the between country differences in incidence.

Hill (1985; 1987; 1989; 1990) has discussed the mechanisms involved in the development of colon cancer including the evidence from animal and metabolic studies which support a role for both saturated and unsaturated fats in the promotion of the disease in animal models. In both animal (Reddy, 1981), and human studies (Hill, 1977; Reddy, 1981) high fat diets increase the excretion of faecal bile acids (Cummings *et al.*, 1978; Hill, 1971) and increased concentrations of faecal bile acids are found in populations with higher rates of colon cancer.

Cancers of the gastrointestinal tract are perhaps those in which diet is most likely to be changed as the disease progresses. The dietary changes may be subtle and not necessarily recognized by the patient and in case-control studies bias may be introduced as the patient will report their current diet rather than pre-illness diet. It is possible therefore that prospective studies will give better information. However, data from prospective studies has so far been inconsistent, possibly due to the limited measures used for dietary assessment (Willet *et al.*, 1990). In a large study of Seventh Day Adventists (Morgan *et al.*, 1988) those in the highest third of fat intake had a higher risk than those in the lowest. Colon cancer has been associated with intakes of processed meat in Norway (Bjelke, 1971) and meat in Sweden (Gerhardsson *et al.*, 1988) and it is possible that this may be associated with its fat content.

In the most recently reported prospective study of 88,751 women 150 cases of colon cancer were identified after 6 years of follow-up. Animal fat was positively associated with the risk of colon cancer after correction for total energy intake; there were also positive correlations for beef, pork and lamb when those eating it daily were compared with those eating it only once per month. Consumption of processed meats and liver was also associated with higher risk but consumption of fish and chicken without skin was associated with decreased risk. The authors also looked at the associations between fat and fibre intake and found that those with the highest fat intake tended to eat less dietary fibre. If those with the lowest fibre and highest fat intakes were compared with those with the highest fibre and lowest fat intakes the relative risk was 2.52. The authors concluded that the highest risk appears to be from animal fat consumption although they did not rule out the fact that the association with meat could be due to other factors such as nitrosamine formation or carcinogens produced on cooking meat.

Whatever the cause their data supports the idea of using less red meat in the diet, replacing this with fish and poultry and making up the lost energy with foods rich in starch and dietary fibre – i.e. the standard low-fat regimen which is being recommended in many countries at the current time. It is unlikely that this type of diet will be harmful unless carried to extremes and it is possible that it may be of benefit in many ways.

Conclusions

As with other theories regarding diet and the aetiology of disease there is now such a wealth of literature relating dietary fat and various cancers that enthusiasts could choose papers to support or refute the idea that high intakes of fat or types of fat are detrimental depending on their viewpoint. However, there are potentially many benefits to be had from a moderate reduction in fat intake. At present it is unclear just how low the intake of fat should be but a reduction to a level supplying 30% of the daily energy intake by those consuming the higher levels common in Northern Europe should not be detrimental if it can be achieved. In Southern Europe there are those who would argue that consuming 40% or more of energy from fat is not detrimental providing that the majority of this is in the form of mono-unsaturated fatty acids (Trichopoulou – this volume). However, there seems to be insufficient data at present to make recommendations about the type of fatty acids which should be consumed apart from the advice to keep saturated fat intake to a maximum of 10–15% energy.

References

Armstrong B, Doll R (1975). Environmental factors and cancer incidence and mortality in different countries with special reference to dietary practices. *Int J Cancer* **15**: 617–631.

Berrino F, Panico S, Muti P (1989). Dietary fat, nutritional status and endocrine related cancers. In *Diet and the aetiology of cancer* (ed Miller AB); Springer-Verlag, Berlin, pp 3–12.

Berta JL, Coste T, Rauteureau J *et al*. (1985). Diet and rectocolonic cancers: results of a case-control study. *Gastroenterol Clin Biol* **9**:L 348–353.

Bjelke E (1980). International Congress Series no 484. Vol 5 of Advances in Tumour Prevention, detection and characterization. In Human cancer: its characterization and treatment (eds Davis W, Harrap KR, Stathopoulos G); Amsterdam Excerpta Medica, pp 158–174.

Bristol JB, Emmett PM, Heaton KW *et al*. (1985). Sugar, fat and fibre and risk of colorectal cancer. *BMJ* **291**: 1467–1470.

Byers T, Marshall J, Graham S *et al*. (1983). A case-control study of dietary and non-dietary factors in cancer. *JNCI* **71**: 681–686.

Carroll KK (1985). Diet and breast cancer – Experimental appoaches. In *Diet and Human Carcinogenesis* (eds Joosens J, Hill MJ, Geboers J); Excerpta Medica Amsterdam, pp 265–275.

Carroll KK, Braden LM, Bell JR, Kalamegham R (1986). Fat and cancer. *Cancer* **58**: 1818–1825.

Chan PC, Cohen L (1975). Dietary fat and growth promotion of rat mammary tumours. *Cancer Res* **35**: 3384–3386.

COMA (1991). Dietary Reference Values for Food Energy and Nutrients for the United Kingdom. Report on Health and Social Subjects 41. London HMSO.

Cramer DW (1989). Lactase persistence and milk consumption as determinants of ovarian cancer risk. *Am J Epidemiol* **130**: 909-910.

Cramer DW, Welch WR, Hutchinson DB *et al*. (1984). Dietary animal fat in relation to ovarian cancer risk. *Obstet Gynecol* **63**: 833-838.

Cramer DW, Harlow BL, Willet WC *et al*. (1989). Galactose consumption and metabolism in relation to the risk of ovarian cancer. *Lancet* **2**: 66–71.

Cummings JH, Wiggins H, Jenkins D *et al*. (1978). The influence of different levels of dietary fat intake on faecal composition, microflora and transit time. *J Clin Invest* **61**: 953–961.

Doll R, Peto R (1981). The causes of cancer: quantitative estimates of avoidable risks of cancer in the United States today. *J Natl Cancer Inst* **66**: 1203–1233.

Donn AS, Muir CS (1985). Prostatic cancer: some epidemiological features. *Bull Cancer* (Paris) **72**: 381–390.

Drasar BS, Irving D (1973). Environmental factors and cancer of the colon and breast. *Brit J Cancer* **27**: 167–172.

Goodwin PJ, Boyd NF (1987). Critical appraisal of the evidence that dietary fat intake is related to breast cancer risk in humans. *JNCI* **79**: 473–485.

Geboers J, Joosens JV, Carroll KK (1985). Introductory remarks to the concensus statement on provisional dietary guidelines. In *Diet and Human Carcinogenesis* (eds Joosens JV, Hill MJ, Geboers J); Excerpta Medica, Amsterdam, pp 337–342.

Gerhardsson M, Floderus B, Norell SE (1988). Physical activity and colon cancer risk. *Int J Epidemiol* **17**: 743–746.

Graham S, Marshall J, Mettlin C *et al.* (1982). Diet in the epidemiology of breast cancer. *Am J Epidemiol* **112**: 68–75.

Graham S, Marshall J, Haughey B *et al.* (1988). Dietary epidemiology of cancer of the colon in western New York. *Am J Epidemiol* **128**: 490–501.

Haenszel W, Berg J, Segi M *et al.* (1973). Large bowel cancer in Hawaiian Japanese. *J Natl Cancer Inst* **51**: 1765–1779.

Henderson BE, Ross R, Bernstein L (1988). Estrogens as a cause of human cancer. *Cancer Res* **48**: 246–253.

Heshmat MY, Kaul L, Kovi J *et al.* (1985). Nutrition and prostate cancer: a case control study. *The prostate* **6**: 7–17.

Hill MJ (1971). The effect of some factors on the faecal concentration of acid steroids, neutral steroids and urobilinogens. *J Path* **104**: 239–245.

Hill MJ (1977). In *Origins of Human Cancer* (eds Hiatt HH, Watson JD, Winstein JA); Cold Springer Harbour, NY: Cold Spring Harbour Laboratory, p1627–1640.

Hill MJ (1985). Mechanisms of colo-rectal carcinogenesis. In *Diet and Human Carcinogenesis* (eds Joosens J, Hill MJ, Geboers J); Excerpta Medica Amsterdam, pp 149–163.

Hill MJ (1987). Dietary fat and human cancer (Review). *Anticancer Research* **7**: 281–292.

Hill MJ (1989). In *Diet and the Aetiology of Cancer* (ed Miller AB) Springer – Verlag, Berlin, Heidelberg, New York, pp 31-38.

Hill MJ (1990). Mode of action of lipids in human carcinogenesis. In *Lipids and Health* (ed Ziant G); Elsevier, pp 19–26.

Hill MJ, Crowther JS, Drasar BS *et al.* (1971). Bacteria and aetiology of cancer of the large bowel. *Lancet* **1**: 95–100.

Hill P, Wynder EL, Garbaczewski L *et al.* (1979). Diet and menarche in different ethnic groups. *Cancer Research* **39**: 5101-5105.

Hirayama T (1985). Diet and cancer: Feasibility and importance of prospective cohort study. In *Diet and Human Carcinogenesis* (eds Joosens J, Hill MJ, Geboers J); Excerpta Medica Amsterdam, pp 191–198.

Hirohata T, Shigematsu T, Nomura A (1985). Occurrence of breast cancer in relation to diet and reproductive history: a case control study in Kukuoka, Japan. *Natl Cancer Inst Monogr* **69**: 187–190.

Hirohata T, Nomura MY, Hankin JH *et al.* (1987). An epidemiological study on the association between diet and breast cancer. *JNCI* **78**: 595–600.

Hislop TG, Coldman AJ, Elwood JM *et al.* (1986). Childhood and recent eating patterns and risk of breast cancer. *Cancer Detect prev* **9**: 47–58.

Howe GR (1985). The use of polytomous dual response data to increase power in case control studies: an application to the association between dietary fat and cancer. *J Chron Dis* **38**: 663-670.

Jain M, Cook GM, Davis FG *et al*. (1980). A case-control study of diet and colo-rectal cancer. *Int J Cancer* **26**: 757–768.

Jenson OM (1985). The role of diet in colo-rectal cancer. In *Diet and Human Carcinogenesis* (eds Joosens J, Hill MJ, Geboers J); Excerpta Medica Amsterdam, pp 137–148.

Jensen OM, Ewertz M, Tjonneland A (1990). Dietary fat and cancer of hormone dependent organs and the pancreas. In *Lipids and Health* (ed Ziant G); Elsevier, pp 73–83.

Jones DY, Schatzkin A, Green SB *et al*. (1987). Dietary fat and breast cancer in the National Health and Nutrition Examination survey. *JNCI* **79**: 465–471.

Katsouyanni K, Trichopoulos D, Boyle P *et al*. (1986). Diet and breast cancer: a case-control study in Greece. *Int J Cancer* **38**: 815–820.

Kinlen LJ (1982). Meat and fat consumption and cancer mortality: a study of a strict religious order in Britain. *Lancet* **1**: 946-949.

Knekt P, Albanes D, Seppanen R *et al*. (1990). Dietary fat and risk of breast cancer. *Am J Clin Nutr* **52**: 903–908.

Kune GA, Kune S (1987). The nutritional causes of colon cancer. *Nutr Cancer* **9**: 1–4.

Le MG, Moulton LH, Hill C *et al*. (1986). Consumption of dairy produce and alcohol in a case-control study of breast cancer. *JNCI* **76**: 49–60.

Lew EA, Garfinkel L (1979). Variations in mortality by weight among 750,000 men and women. *J Chron Dis* **32**: 563–576.

Lubin F, Wax Y, Modan B (1986). Role of fat, animal protein and dietary fiber intake in breast cancer etiology. *JNCI* **76**: 685-689.

Lubin JH, Burns PE, Blot WJ *et al*. (1981). Dietary factors and breast cancer risk. *Int J Cancer* **28**: 685–689.

Lyon JL, Mahoney AW, West DW *et al*. (1987). Energy intake: its relationship to colon cancer risk. *J Natl Cancer Inst* **78**: 557-569.

Macquart-Moulin G, Riboli E, Cornee J *et al*. (1986). Case-control study on colorectal cancer and diet in Marseilles. *Int J Cancer* **38**: 183–191.

Marr JW, Heady JA (1986). Within and between-person variation in dietary surveys: number of days needed to classify individuals. *Human Nutr Appl Nutr* **40A**: 347–364.

McMahon B (1974). Risk factors for endometrial cancer. *Gynaecol Oncol* **2**: 122–129.

Mettlin C (1986). Methodological issues in epidemiologic studies of dietary fat and cancer. In *Dietary Fat and Cancer* (eds Ip C, Birt DF, Rogers AE, Mettlin C); Alan R Liss, New York. pp 3–16.

Mettlin CJ, Piver S (1990). A case-control study of milk drinking and ovarian cancer risk. *Am J Epidemiol* **132**: 871–876.

Miller AB, Kelly A, Choi NW *et al*. (1978). A study of diet and breast cancer. *Am J Epidemiol* **127**: 440–453.

Mills PK, Annegers JF, Phillips RL (1988). Animal product consumption and subsequent fatal breast cancer risk among Seventh day Adventists. *Am J Epidemiol* **127**: 440–453.

Mishina T, Wanatabe H, Araki H *et al.* (1985). Epidemiological study of prostate cancer by matched-pair analysis. *Prostate* **6**: 423–436.

Morgan JW, Fraser GE, Phillips RL *et al.* (1988). Dietary factors and colon cancer incidence among Seventh-day Adventists. *Am J Epidemiol* **128**: 918 Abst.

Muir C, Waterhouse J, Mack T *et al.* (1987). Cancer incidence in five continents. Vol V IARC Scientific Publication No 88. International Agency for Research on Cancer, Lyon, 1987.

Nomura A, Henderson BE, Lee J (1978). Breast cancer and diet among the Japanese in Hawaii. *Am J Clin Nutr* **31**: 2020–2050.

Phillips RL (1975). Role of lifestyle and dietary habits in risk of cancer among Seventh-day Adventists: preliminary results. *Cancer Research* **35**: 3513–3522.

Potter JD (1987). Letter. *N Engl Med J* **317**: p166.

Potter JD, McMichael AJ (1986). Diet and cancer of the colon and rectum: a case-control study. *J Natl Cancer Inst* **76**: 557–69.

Prentice RL, Pepe M, Self GS (1989). Dietary fat and breast cancer: a quantitative assessment of the epidemiological literature and a discussion of methodological issues. *Cancer Res* **49**: 3147–3156.

Reddy BS (1981). Diet and excretion of bile acids. *Cancer Res* **41**: 3766–8.

Ries W (1973). Feeding behaviour in obesity. *Proc Nut Soc* **32**: 187.

Rohan TE, McMicheal AJ, Baghurst PA (1987). A population-based case-control study of diet and breast cancer in Australia. *Am J Epidemiol* **128**: 478–498.

Rose DP, Boyer AP, Synde EL (1986). International comparisons of mortality rates for cancer of the breast, ovary, prostate and colon. *Cancer* **58**: 2363–2371.

Sarin R, Tandon RK, Paul S *et al.* (1985). Diet, body fat and plasma lipids in breast cancer. *Indian J Med Res* **81**: 493–498.

Slattery ML, Schumacher MC, Smith KR *et al.* (1988). Physical activity, diet and risk of colon cancer in Utah. *Am J Epidemiol* **128**: 989–999.

Talamini R, La Vechhia C, De Carli A (1984). Social factors, diet and breast cancer in a Northern Italian population. *Br J Cancer* **49**: 723–729.

Tuyns AJ, Haelterman M, Kaaks R (1987). Colorectal cancer and the intake of nutrients: oligosaccharides are a risk factor, fats are not: a case-control study in Belgium. *Nutr Cancer* **10**: 181-196.

Thomas DB, Chu J (1986). Nutritional and endocrine factors in reproductive organ cancers: Opportunities for primary prevention. *J Chron Dis* **12**: 1031–1050.

Whitemore AF, Wu-Williams AH, Lee M *et al.* (1990). Diet, physical activity and colon cancer among Chinese in North America and China. *J Natl Cancer Inst* **82**: 915–926.

Willet WC, McMahon B (1984). Diet and cancer – an overview. *New Engl J Med* **310**: 633–638.

Willet WC, Stampfer MJ (1986). Total energy intake: implications for epidemiologic analyses. *Am J Epidemiol* **124**: 17–27.

Willet WC, Stampfer MJ, Colditz GA *et al.* (1987). Dietary fat and the risk of breast cancer *N Engl J Med* **316**: 22–28.

Willet WC, Meir J, Stampner MD *et al.* (1990). Relation of meat, fat and fiber intake to the risk of colon cancer. Prospective study among women. *New Engl J Med* **323**: 1664–1672.

Wynder EL, Rose DP, Cohen LA (1986). Diet and breast cancer in causation and therapy. *Cancer* **58:** 1804–1813.

Wynder EL, Mabuchi K, Whitmore WF (1971). Epidemiology of cancer of the prostate. *Cancer* **28:** 344–360.

La Vechhia C, Decarli A, Fascoli M *et al.* (1986). Nutrition and diet in the aetiology of endometrial cancer. *Cancer* **57:** 1248-1253.

Zaridze DG (1983). Environmental etiology of large bowel cancer. *J Natl Cancer Inst* **70:** 389–400.

Zemla B (1985). The role of selected dietary elements in breast cancer risk among native and migrant populations in Poland. *Nutr Cancer* **6:** 187–190.

CHAPTER 12

Alcohol and Cancer

S FRANCESCHI

Epidemiology Unit
Aviano Cancer Center, Via Pedemontana Occ, 33081 Aviano (PN), Italy

Introduction

Epidemiological studies have demonstrated that alcohol interacts with tobacco smoke in the development of cancers of oral cavity, pharynx and oesophagus (Blot *et al.*, 1988; Ferraroni *et al.*, 1989; IARC, 1988; La Vecchia *et al.*, 1986; Tuyns *et al.*, 1988; Tuyns *et al.*, 1977). How the effects of alcohol result in increased risk for cancer of different sites is not well understood and several mechanisms can be envisaged (IARC, 1988; Doll and Peto, 1981; Fraumeni, 1979; McCoy and Wynder, 1979; Tuyns, 1979). Firstly, alcohol may function as a solvent, thus facilitating the passage of carcinogens through cellular membranes. This mechanism, however, does not explain increase in cancer risk in body areas which do not come into direct contact with it. Secondly, ethanol consumption leads to an enhancement in the liver drug-metabolising capability in both humans and experimental animals and may, therefore, activate carcinogenic substances. In this particular mechanism, it remains to explain the reason for the high site-specificity of the alcohol effect, since all tissues in the body would be exposed to the results of changes in liver metabolism. Conversely, after the onset of alcohol-induced cirrhosis, a decreased ability to detoxify carcinogens may cause an increase in their systemic concentration. Furthermore, ethanol consumption may alter intracellular metabolism of the epithelial cells at the target site. Such impairment of cellular function (i.e. decreased mitochondrial function, increased DNA alkylation, etc) can be aggravated by the coexistence of nutritional deficiencies (including niacin, riboflavin, iron, etc) (Day, 1984; Darby *et al.*, 1975; Decarli *et al.*, 1987; Li *et al.*, 1989; Lu *et al.*, 1985; McLaughlin *et al.*, 1988; Rossing *et al.*, 1989; Van Rensburg, 1986; Wahrendorf *et al.*, 1989). Finally, it must not be overlooked that the concentration of ethanol attained in humans at least in the upper digestive tract can cause local irritation.

115

In the present review the association of alcohol consumption with risk of cancer with special emphasis on tumours of the upper digestive tract (i.e. oral cavity, pharynx and oesophagus), will be examined. Large parts of the data are derived from a case-control study, ongoing in the Northern part of Italy since 1985, which includes approximately 600 cases of cancer of the upper digestive tract and twice as many hospital controls with acute illnesses other than tumours or any condition known to be related to alcohol and tobacco consumption (Franceschi *et al.*, 1990; Talamini *et al.*, 1990; La Vecchia and Negri, 1989; Barra *et al.*, 1990). This investigation, on account of the high alcohol intake and social acceptability of chronic heavy drinking in the study area, and the elevated prevalence of alcohol-related disease (Franceschi *et al.*, 1989) offered a special opportunity to further explore several open issues, such as the role of various types of alcoholic beverages and the effect of alcohol in the absence of smoking.

The Effect of Alcohol

The alcohol-related risks for cancers of the oral cavity, pharynx and oesophagus, adjusted for tobacco, are shown in Table 1 (Franceschi *et al.*, 1990). A highly significant direct trend in risk with an increasing number of drinks of wine consumed emerged for each cancer site. Significantly elevated risks, however, became apparent only in those who drank 56 or more glasses of wine per week (about 1 litre per day). Odds ratios (ORs) of 8.5, 10.9, and 14.0 for cancer of the oral cavity, pharynx and oesophagus, respectively, were seen among those persons who reported drinking 84 or more glasses of wine per week. Total alcohol intake mostly reflected wine consumption and, in a similar way, showed for heavy drinkers (60 or more drinks per week) the most elevated OR for oesophageal cancer (OR = 6.0). Conversely, the duration of the alcohol-drinking habit did not appear to be related to risks for any of the upper digestive tract tumours considered here.

The joint effect of tobacco and alcohol intake is examined in Table 2 (Franceschi, 1990). Cases of oral cavity and pharyngeal cancer are considered together; also abstainers and light alcohol drinkers (<34 drinks per week) are combined since the associated ORs (Table 1) appeared to be very similar. The risk of oral cavity and pharyngeal cancer for the highest levels of alcohol and smoking was increased 80-fold relative to the lowest levels of both factors. The joint effect of smoking and drinking appeared, thereafter, greater than multiplicative. For oesophageal cancer, combined high levels of alcohol and cigarette consumption increased the risk 18 times over the risk for the lowest levels of consumption. The pattern of combined risk for this site appears to be intermediate between additive and multiplicative. The effect of drinking in non-smokers was only slightly stronger

Table 1 Odds ratios of cancer of the oral cavity, pharynx and oesophagus in males according to alcohol drinking habits[a] – Northern Italy

	Odds ratio[b] (95% confidence interval)		
	Oral cavity (n=157)	Pharynx (n=134)	Oesophagus (n=288)
Wine (drinks/wk)			
≤20[c]	1	1	1
21–34	1.1(0.5–2.3)	0.7(0.3–1.6)	1.2(0.8–1.8)
35–55	1.9(0.9–3.7)	1.9(0.9–3.7)	1.9(1.2–3.0)
56–83	4.9(2.6–9.5)	3.1(1.6–6.1)	4.4(2.8–6.9)
84+	8.5(3.6–20.2)	10.9(4.7–25.3)	14.0(6.4–30.6)
χ^2_1 (trend)	47.68[d]	46.44[d]	66.79[d]
Beer (drinks/wk)			
0[c]	1	1	1
1–13	1.0(0.6–1.8)	0.5(0.3–1.0)	1.1(0.6–1.6)
14+	0.8(0.5–1.4)	0.9(0.5–1.5)	1.8(1.2–2.8)
χ^2_1 (trend)	0.30	0.47	5.25[e]
Hard liquors (drinks/wk)			
0[c]	1	1	1
1–6	0.7(0.4–1.3)	0.4(0.2–0.9)	0.8(0.5–1.3)
7+	0.9(0.6–1.3)	1.2(0.8–1.8)	1.8(1.3–2.6)
χ^2_1 (trend)	0.66	0.24	9.58[d]
Total (drinks/wk)			
≤19[c]	1	1	1
20–34	1.1(0.5–2.5)	0.9(0.4–2.0)	1.0(0.6–1.7)
35–59	3.2(1.6–6.2)	1.5(0.8–3.1)	3.1(2.0–4.7)
60+	3.4(1.7–7.1)	3.6(1.8–7.2)	6.0(3.7–10.0)
χ^2_1(trend)	18.74[d]	21.66[d]	68.37[d]

[a] Total sample size varies with the number of cases and controls with incomplete information.
[b] Estimates from logistic regression adjusted for age, area of residence, years of education, occupation and smoking habits.
[c] Reference category.
[d] $p<0.01$
[e] $p<0.05$

Table 2 Odds ratio[a] of cancers of the oral cavity/pharynx and oesophagus in males according to smoking and alcohol drinking habits – Northern Italy

Smoking[b] status	Odds ratio Alcohol intake (total drinks per week)			Total[c]
	< 35	35–39	≥60	
Oral cavity/pharynx				
(n=291)				
Non-smokers	1	1.6	2.3	1
Light	3.1	5.4	10.9	3.7
Intermediate	10.9	26.6	36.4	14.1
Heavy	17.6	40.2	79.6	25.0
Total[d]	1	2.3	3.4	
Oesophagus				
(n-288)				
Non-smokers	1	0.8	7.9	1
Light	1.1	7.9	9.4	2.5
Intermediate	2.7	8.8	16.7	4.0
Heavy	6.4	11.0	17.5	6.6
Total[d]	1	3.1	5.7	

a   Estimates from logistic regression adjusted for age, area of residence, years of education, occupation, drinks per week and smoking habits.
b   Smoking status defined in four categories: (1) non-smokers; (2) light, ex-smokers who quit ≥10 years ago; or smokers of 1–14 cigarettes/day for <30 years; (3) intermediate, 15–24 cigarettes/day regardless of duration, 30–39 years duration regardless of amount, 1–24 cigarettes/day for ≥40 years, or ≥15 cigarettes/day for <30 years; (4) heavy smokers of ≥25 cigarettes/day for ≥40 years.
c   Estimates from logistic regression adjusted for age, area of residence, years of education, occupation and drinks per week.
d   Estimates from logistic regression adjusted for age, area of residence, years of education, occupation and smoking habits.

than the effect of smoking in light drinkers (OR = 7.9 vs 6.4). Thus, at variance with cancer of the oral cavity and pharynx, where the ORs for tobacco are appreciably higher than those of alcohol, alcohol appears to have an effect on the risk of oesophageal cancer approximately as strong as smoking.

Alcohol in Non-smokers

Table 3 considers the risk of oral and pharyngeal cancer related to alcohol among non-smokers (Talamini *et al.*, 1990). There was a trend toward increasing risk with increasing alcohol consumption (age- and sex-adjusted χ^2 for trend = 4.08; p = 0.04). Whereas among males no difference was seen between abstainers and moderate drinkers, among females an elevated risk emerged also for those who drank fewer than 14 drinks per week. Overall ORs for ≤14 and ≥56 drinks per week were 1.5 and 2.2, respectively. Twenty-one out of twenty-five non-smoking cases and 298/519 non-smoking controls who described themselves as drinkers reported drinking only wine. All cases and 98% of controls said they drank wine predominantly.

These results on the effect of alcohol in 27 lifetime non-smoker cases of oral and pharyngeal cancer and 572 non-smoker controls (Talamini *et al.*, 1990) represent a contribution to a debate which is still open. Due to insufficient numbers of non-smoker cancer cases, in many previous investigations, non-smokers and light smokers (i.e. <10 cigarettes per day) had to be combined (Graham *et al.*, 1977; Olsen *et al.*, 1985; De Stefani *et al.*, 1988; Merletti *et al.*, 1989) thus making it difficult to interpret the 2- to 20-fold increased risk of oral and pharyngeal cancer in those individuals who reported variously defined heavy alcohol consumption.

Table 3 Odds ratios in never-smoker cases of oral and pharyngeal cancer and never-smoker controls by alcohol consumption and sex – Northern Italy

Weekly alcohol consumption (drinks/week)	Males Cases	Controls	Females Cases	Controls	Odds ratio (95% confidence interval)[a]
0	1	27	1	97 }	
				}	1[b]
<14	–	28	9	70 }	
14–55	3	191	11	115	1.5 (0.6–3.7)
>55	2	42	–	2	2.2 (0.2–27.9)
χ^2_1 (trend)					4.08 p = 0.04

[a] Mantel-Haenszel estimates adjusted for age and sex.
[b] Reference category.

Among those investigators who have been able to report on alcohol-related risk in strictly defined non-smokers, Wynder *et al.* (1957) found no difference in drinking habits among 16 cases of cancer of the oral cavity and pharynx and nine controls who did not smoke, while an approximate doubling of risk was seen by Rothman and Keller (Rothman and Keller, 1972) and Elwood *et al.* (1984) among non-smokers who consumed approximately 300 grams of alcohol per week. Also Tuyns *et al.* (1988), in a large study which showed an effect of alcohol of pharyngeal cancer risk across all strata of smoking habits, were able to report on only 9 cases of lifetime non-smokers with tumour of the hypopharynx or epilarynx (and in whom they found higher alcohol consumption than among controls). Blot *et al.* (1988) observed a trend toward increasing risk with drinking among 50 non-smoking male cases of oral and pharyngeal cancer (OR for ≥30 drinks per week = 5.8). Their suggestion that lower risks may be associated with intake of wine compared to liquor or beer are, however, not supported by the present study in which, at variance with the US data, virtually all drinkers drank wine predominantly and two thirds drank wine only.

Table 4 shows the effect of alcohol consumption on risk of cancer of the oesophagus in non-smokers (La Vecchia and Negri, 1989). There was no difference in risk between abstainers and moderate drinkers (<4 drinks per day, about 50 g of pure ethanol, combined in Table 4 in the reference

Table 4 Odds ratios in never-smoker cases of cancer of the oesophagus and never-smoker controls by alcohol consumption and sex – Northern Italy

Weekly alcohol consumption (drinks/week)	Males		Females		Odds ratio (95% confidence interval)[a]
	Cases	Controls	Cases	Controls	
0	2	26	8	77 }	
				}	1[b]
<28	3	90	14	114 }	
28–55	3	66	4	9	2.1 (0.8–5.3)
≥55	3	21	1	1	3.6 (0.9–13.6)
χ_1^2 (trend)					6.09 ($p=0.01$)

[a] Mantel-Haenszel estimates adjusted for age and sex.
[b] Reference category.

category in order to give more stable estimates), but the risk increased markedly for higher levels of alcohol consumption. The point estimates were 2.1 for 4 to 8 drinks per day and 3.6 for over 8 drinks per day, with a clear dose–effect relation and a significant trend in risk ($p = 0.01$).

These results (La Vecchia and Negri, 1989), therefore, confirm the findings of a study from Calvados, France (Tuyns, 1983), which included a sufficient number of non-smokers to show a substantial effect of alcohol alone, but in which the number of non-drinking smokers (11 males) was probably too small to provide reliable estimates for tobacco alone.

Finally, in order to confirm further the independent effects of alcohol in upper digestive tract carcinogenesis, it is worth noting that the ORs for alcohol in non-smokers (Talamini *et al.*, 1990; La Vecchia and Negri, 1989) were very similar to those emerging from the overall data set, after adjustment for smoking and drinking habits, respectively (Table 1) (Franceschi *et al.*, 1990).

In conclusion, tobacco does not seem to be a requisite co-factor for alcohol-related cancers.

Type of Alcoholic Beverage

Table 5 shows the distribution of oral and pharyngeal cancers and controls according to different drinking patterns (Barra *et al.*, 1990). Moderate drinkers (i.e. ≤55 drinks/week) did not show a significant elevation of cancer risk regardless of which type(s) of alcoholic beverage were consumed. Increased ORs clearly emerged in heavy and very heavy (i.e. ≥84 drinks/week) drinkers which, although ranging from 4.1 for drinkers of a combination of wine, beer and spirits to 11.2 for drinkers of wine only, were not statistically heterogeneous.

A very similar risk pattern emerged with respect to cancer of the oesophagus, where ORs for moderate drinkers tended to be low (ORs from 1.7 to 2.5) and either non-significant or of borderline statistical significance. The elevation of ORs in heavy and very heavy drinkers (ORs from 6.0 to 15.0) appeared also to be substantially independent of the type(s) of alcoholic beverage habitually consumed. The aforementioned tendency of individuals who reported consumption of wine only to show higher risk increases when compared to individuals who consumed combinations of alcoholic beverages was seen in oesophageal cancer as well (Table 6).

Since wine consumption was very common in the present series and virtually no heavy or very heavy drinkers described themselves as consumers of beer and/or spirit only, such categories had to be grouped both for oral and pharyngeal cancer and oesophageal cancer, thus providing an estimate of risk which did not compare well with the others.

Table 5 Odds ratios of cancer of the oral cavity and pharynx according to type(s) of alcoholic beverage consumed – Northern Italy

Types of beverage	Number of cases: Number of controls [a]			Odds ratio[b,c] (95% confidence interval)		
	Alcohol intake (drinks/week)			Alcohol intake (drinks/week)		
	≤55	56–83	≥84	≤55	56–83	≥84
Wine only	44:412	48:84	14:8	1.9 (1.0–3.4)	7.3 (3.8–14.1)	11.2 (3.8–33.1)
Wine & beer	3:58	13:27	21:20	0.7 (0.2–2.5)	3.9 (1.6–9.6)	7.4 (3.2–17.3)
Wine & spirits	13:26	34:4	32:5	1.1 (0.5–2.4)	3.5 (1.7–6.9)	9.9 (4.3–22.7)
Beer only	3:40	–:5	1:1 }			
Spirits only	2:68	–:–	–:– }	0.8 (0.3–2.0)		
Beer & spirits	1:26	1:4	–:5 }			
All three	5:66	12:58	41:66	0.8 (0.3–2.3)	1.8 (0.8–4.4)	4.1 (2.0–8.2)

a   Total sample size varies with the number of cases and controls with incomplete information.
b   Estimates from multiple logistic regression equations including terms for age, area of residence, occupation, smoking and drinking habits.
c   Seventeen cases and 386 controls who were either abstainer or drinker of ≤20 glasses of wine/week were used as reference category.

Some studies have attempted to estimate the effect of specific beverages on the upper digestive tract. The results of these studies are in agreement with the possibility that all types of beverage contribute to cancer risk in proportion to their alcoholic content. A predominant role of spirits in oral, pharyngeal and oesophageal cancer causation has, however, emerged in some instances. Wynder *et al.* (1957) reported higher relative risks for oral cancer among whisky drinkers when compared to beer and/or wine drinkers. They failed, however, to find very heavy drinkers among individuals who abstained from whisky. Higher proportions of drinkers of whisky, beer or combinations of these, but not of wine only, were found among cases of cancer of the oral cavity and pharynx by Keller and Terris (1965) in a case-control study in New York City. Williams and Horm (1977) found similar risk estimates in alcohol drinkers, regardless of the type of beverage, in a study from the United States Third National Survey, while Kabat

Table 6 Odds ratios of cancer of the oesophagus according to type(s) of alcoholic beverage consumed – Northern Italy

Types of beverage	Number of cases: Number of controls [a]			Odds ratio [b,c] (95% confidence interval)		
	Alcohol intake (drinks/week)			Alcohol intake (drinks/week)		
	≤55	56–83	≥84	≤55	56–83	≥84
Wine only	61:412	39:84	7:8	1.7 (1.1–2.7)	5.4 (3.1–9.3)	15.0 (4.6–49.1)
Wine & beer	6:58	8:27	6:20	1.8 (0.7–4.5)	4.3 (1.6–11.3)	4.3 (1.5–12.4)
Wine & spirits	27:177	31:98	11:19	1.8 (1.0–3.1)	3.6 (2.0–6.4)	10.0 (4.1–24.5)
Beer only	5:40	–:5	–:1 }			
Spirits only	8:68	–:–	–:– }	1.6 (0.8–3.0)		
Beer & spirits	–:26	4:4	–:5 }			
All three	9:66	13:51	18:66	2.5 (1.1–6.0)	5.0 (2.3–10.9)	6.0 (2.9–12.3)

a   Total sample size varies with the number of cases and controls with incomplete information.
b   Estimates from multiple logistic regression equations including terms for age, area of residence, occupation, smoking and drinking habits.
c   Seventeen cases and 386 controls who were either abstainer or drinker of ≤20 glasses of wine/week were used as reference category.

and Wynder (1989) reported increased risks only in drinkers of beer and whisky. In a large population based study of oral and pharyngeal cancer conducted in four areas of the US (Blot *et al..*, 1988) the trends were strongest for consumption of beer and spirits and persisted after adjustment of one for the other. Conversely, there was little or no excess risk for wine drinkers of up to 5 drinks/day.

In a cohort of Danish brewery workers, beer appeared to exert the strongest effect on causation of oesophageal cancer (Jensen, 1979). Similar suggestions concerning a predominant effect of beer came also from the United States (Mashberg *et al.*, 1981; Mettlin *et al.*, 1981; Graham *et al.*, 1990) and South Africa (Segal *et al.*, 1988).

In an area of Northern France with very high cider intake, Tuyns *et al.* (1977; 1979) reported the specific role played by cider and apple jack (distillates of apple cider) in the aetiology of oesophageal cancer. However, in the same country, no significant increases in risk for the oral cavity and pharynx were reported by Leclerc *et al.* (1987) for any alcoholic beverage, including cider. In Latin American Countries, Martinez (1969) and De Stefani *et al.* (1988) found no differences in the deleterious effects of red wine, beer and hard liquors on the causation of oral and pharyngeal cancer.

According to the data in Table 5 and 6, ORs both for cancer of the oral cavity and pharynx and for oesophageal cancer, (alcohol intake being equal) tended to be lower in those individuals who described themselves as habitual drinkers of two or three types of alcoholic beverage, as compared to drinkers of wine only (Barra *et al.*, 1990). Such heterogeneity, however, in addition to not being statistically significant, can probably be explained by the tendency of self reports to underestimate alcohol intake, particularly at high levels of consumption (Boland and Roizen, 1973).

As shown by questionnaire-based dietary studies (Pietinen *et al.*, 1988) as well as investigations on smokers who used a variety of kinds of tobacco (Doll and Peto, 1976), the possibility of reporting different sources of relevant exposure (e.g. wine, beer and/or spirits) may well have reduced the phenomenon of under-reporting among drinkers of combinations of alcoholic beverages in respect to drinkers of wine only.

In conclusion, the results from the aforementioned study (Barra *et al.*, 1990) from the Northern part of Italy, an area with very high wine intake, confirm that wine *per se* can cause very large excesses of tumours of the oral cavity, pharynx and oesophagus. It appears, therefore, from this and previous studies that the most frequently used alcoholic beverage in each area tends to emerge, in turn, as the most important determinant of upper digestive tract tumours. In fact, heavy and very heavy drinkers who avoid the consumption of the locally commonest (and consequently cheapest) alcoholic beverages are extremely rare. This suggests that all the various types of alcoholic beverage are carcinogenic and that the apparent differences in the risk estimates of each single study are partly or totally due to different levels and/or sociocultural correlates of drinking patterns in various populations.

Attributable Risk and Conclusions

In terms of attributable risk (Bruzzi *et al.*, 1985) in the context of public health interventions, Blot *et al.* (1988) reported that 80% of the risk for oral cavity and pharyngeal cancer could be attributed to smoking. Tuyns *et al.* (1988) reported attributable risks for alcohol alone of 68% for pharyngeal cancer. The study from North Italy shows attributable risks of over 75% for every site for smoking and alcohol together (Franceschi *et al.*, 1990). Although these factors were moderately correlated in our data, the widespread use of wine as a beverage taken with meals among non-smokers and smokers alike, appears to lead to near independence of smoking and alcohol with respect to the attributable risk of these factors together (Berrino *et al.*, 1988). As expected, smoking showed a higher attributable risk than alcohol for cancers of the oral cavity (76% versus 55%), and pharynx (69% versus 45%). For cancer of the oesophagus, alcohol showed a slightly higher attributable risk than smoking (52% versus 40%).

The observation that the interaction between alcohol and tobacco appears greater than multiplicative for oral and pharyngeal cancer, multiplicative for laryngeal and intermediate between additive and multiplicative for oesophageal cancer finds an interesting potential interpretation in terms of physiology and pattern of exposure to alcohol and tobacco in each of these sites (Franceschi *et al.*, 1990). Oral cavity and pharynx, in fact, are directly exposed to both risk factors, while larynx is directly exposed to tobacco but not to alcohol and oesophagus is directly exposed to alcohol but not to tobacco.

From a public health viewpoint, as noted by a number of investigators (Blot *et al.*, 1988; Franceschi *et al.*, 1990; Saracci, 1987; Flanders and Rothman, 1982), the implication of an interaction between smoking and alcohol which appears to be, on the whole, greater than additive, is a substantial reduction in the occurrence of cancers of the upper digestive tract by eliminating or moderating one or the other of these high risk behaviours.

Finally, it is worth remembering that pure alcohol is not by itself carcinogenic by any of the animal experiments thus far devised (Doll and Peto, 1981). The association between alcohol and cancer of the upper digestive tract is certainly one of the most certain and accurately quantified in the cancer field and its discovery entirely derives from epidemiological data. It constitutes, therefore, one of the most stringent examples of the unwisdom of basing one's beliefs about human cancer too closely on laboratory studies (IARC, 1988; Doll and Peto, 1981).

Acknowledgements

This work was conducted with the contribution of the Italian Association for Research on Cancer and the Italian League against Tumours. We thank Dr Anna E Barón for her useful suggestions and Mrs Anna Redivo for editorial assistance.

References

Barra S, Franceschi S, Negri E, Talamini R, La Vecchia C (1990). Type of alcoholic beverage and cancer of the oral cavity, pharynx and oesophagus in an Italian area with high wine consumption. *Int J Cancer* **46:** 1017–1020.

Berrino F, Merletti F, Zubiri A, Del Moral A, Raymond L, Estève J, Tuyns AJ (1988). A comparative study of smoking, drinking and dietary habits in population samples in France, Italy, Spain and Switzerland. II. Tobacco Smoking. *Rev Epidém Santé Publ* **36:** 166–176.

Blot WJ, McLaughlin JK, Winn DM, Austin DF, Greenberg RS, Preston-Martin S, Bernstein L, Schoenberg JB, Stemhagen A, Fraumeni JF Jr (1988). Smoking and drinking in relation to oral and pharyngeal cancer. *Cancer Res* **48:** 3282–3287.

Boland B, Roizen R (1973). Sales slips and survey responses: new data on the reliability of survey consumption measures. *Drinking Drug Pract Surv* **8:** 5–10.

Breslow NE, Day NE (1980). *Statistical methods in cancer research. The analysis of case-control studies*, Vol I, IARC. Sci Publ No 32, IARC, Lyon.

Breslow NE, Storer BE (1985). General relative risk function for case-control studies. *Am J Epidemiol* **122:** 149–162.

Bruzzi P, Green SB, Byar DP, Brinton LA, Schairer C (1985). Estimating the population attributable risk for multiple risk factors using case-control data. *Am J Epidemiol* **122:** 904–914.

Darby WJ, McNutt KW, Todhunter EN (1975). Niacin. *Nutr Rev* **33:** 289–297.

Day NE (1984). The geographic pathology of cancer of the oesophagus. *Medical Bulletin* **40:** 329–334.

Decarli A, Liati P, Negri E, Franceschi S and La Vecchia C (1987). Vitamin A and other dietary factors in the etiology of esophageal cancer. *Nutr Cancer* **10:** 29–37.

De Stefani E, Correa P, Oreggia F, Deneo-Pellegrini H, Fernandez G, Zavala D, Carzoglio J, Leiva J, Fontham E, Rivero S (1988). Black tobacco, wine and maté in oropharyngeal cancer. A case-control study from Uruguay. *Rev Epidémiol Santé Publique* **36:** 389–394.

Doll R, Peto R (1976). Mortality in relation to smoking: 20 years' observation on male British doctors. *BMJ* **2:** 1525–1536.

Doll R, Peto R (1981). The causes of cancer: quantitative estimates of avoidable risks of cancer in United States today. *J Natl Cancer Inst* **66:** 1191–1308.

Elwood JM, Pearson JCG, Skippen DH, Jackson SM (1984). Alcohol, smoking, social and occupational factors in the aetiology of cancer of the oral cavity, pharynx and larynx. *Int J Cancer* **34:** 603–612.

Feldman JG, Boxer P (1979). Relationship of drinking to head and neck cancer. *Prev Med* **8:** 507–519.

Ferranroni M, Negri E, La Vecchia C, D'Avanzo B, Franceschi S (1989). Socio-economic indicators, tobacco and alcohol in the aetiology of digestive tract neoplasms. *Int J Epidemiol* **18:** 556–562.

Flanders WD, Rothman KJ (1982). Interaction of alcohol and tobacco in laryngeal cancer. *Am J Epidemiol* **115:** 371–379.

Franceschi S, Bidoli E, Barra S, Gerdol D, Serraino D, Talamini R (1989). *Atlante della mortalità per tumori nella Regione Friuli-Venezia Giulia, 1980–1983*, Servizio di Epidemiologia, Centro di Riferimento Oncologico, Aviano, Italy.

Franceschi S, Talamini R, Barra S, Barón AE, Negri E, Bidoli E, Serraino S and La Vecchia C (1990). Smoking and drinking in relation to cancers of the oral cavity, pharynx, larynx and esophagus in Northern Italy. *Cancer Res* **50:** 6502–6507.

Franco EL, Kowalski LP, Oliveira BV, Curado MP, Pereira RN, Silva ME, Fava AS, Torloni H (1989). Risk factors for oral cancer in Brazil: a case-control study. *Int J Cancer* **43:** 992–1000.

Fraumeni JF Jr (1979). Epidemiological opportunities in alcohol-related cancer. *Cancer Res* **39:** 2851–2852.

Graham S, Dayal H, Rohrer T, Swanson M, Sultz H, Shedd D, Fischman S (1977). Dentition, diet, tobacco and alcohol in the epidemiology of oral cancer. *J Natl Cancer Inst* **59:** 1611–1618.

Graham S, Marshall J, Haughey B, Brasure J, Freudenheim J, Zielezny M, Wilkinson G, Nolan J (1990). Nutritional epidemiology of cancer of the esophagus. *Am J Epidemiol* **131:** 454–467.

IARC Working Group on the Evaluation of Carcinogenic Risks to Humans (1988). IARC Monog Eval Carcinog Risks Hum. *Alcohol Drinking* **44:** IARC, Lyon.

Jensen OM (1979). Cancer morbidity and causes of death among Danish Brewery workers. *Int J Cancer* **23:** 454–463.

Kabat GC, Wynder EL (1989). Type of alcoholic beverage and oral cancer. *Int J Cancer* **43:** 190–194.

Keller AZ, Terris M (1965). The association of alcohol and tobacco with cancer of the mouth and pharynx. *Am J Publ Health* **55:** 1578–1585.

La Vecchia C, Liati P, Decarli A, Negrello I, Franceschi S (1986). Tar yields of cigarettes and the risk of oesophageal cancer. *Int J Cancer* **38:** 381–385.

La Vecchia C, Negri E (1989). The role of alcohol in oesophageal cancer in non-smokers and of tobacco in non-drinkers. *Int J Cancer* **43:** 784–785.

Leclerc A, Brugère J, Luce D, Point D, Guenel P (1987). Type of alcoholic beverage and cancer of the upper respiratory and digestive tract. *Eur J Cancer Clin Oncol* **23:** 529–534.

Li J-Y, Ershow AG, Chen Z-J, Wacholder S, Li G-Y, Guo W, Li B, Blot WJ (1989). A case-control study of cancer of the esophagus and gastric cardia in Linxian. *Int J Cancer* **43:** 755–761.

Lu J-B, Yang W-X, Liu J-M, Li Y-S, Qin Y-M (1985). Trends in morbidity and mortality for oesophageal cancer in Linxian Country, 1959–1983. *Int J Cancer* **36:** 643–645.

Martinez I (1969). Factors associated with cancer of the esophagus, mouth and pharynx in Puerto Rico. *J Natl Cancer Inst* **42:** 1069–1094.

Mashberg A, Garfinkel L, Harris S (1981). Alcohol as a primary risk factor in oral squamous carcinoma. *CA* **31:** 146–155.

McCoy GD, Wynder E (1979). Etiological and preventive implications in alcohol carcinogenesis. *Cancer Res* **39:** 2844–2850.

McLaughlin JK, Gridley G, Block G, Winn DM, Preston-Martin S, Shoenberg JB, Greenberg RS, Stemhagen S, Austin DF, Ershow AG, Blot WJ, Fraumeni JF Jr (1988). Dietary factors in oral and pharyngeal cancer. *J Natl Cancer Inst* **80:** 1237–1243.

Merletti F, Boffetta P, Ciccone G, Mashberg A, Terracini B (1989). Role of tobacco and alcoholic beverages in the etiology of cancer of the oral cavity/oropharynx in Torino, Italy. *Cancer Res* **49**: 4919–4924.

Mettlin C, Graham S, Priore R, Marshal J, Swanson M (1981). Diet and cancer of the esophagus. *Nutr Cancer* **2**: 143–147.

Olsen J, Sabroe S, Ipsen J (1985). Effect of combined alcohol and tobacco exposure on risk of cancer of the hypopharynx. *J Epidemiol Community Health* **39**: 304–307.

Pietinen P, Hartman AM, Haapa E, Rasanen L, Haapakoski J, Palmgren J, Albanes D, Virtamo J, Huttunen JK (1988). Reproducibility and validity of dietary assessment instruments. *Am J Epidemiol* **128**: 655–676.

Rossing MA, Vaughan TL, McKnight B (1989). Diet and pharyngeal cancer. *Int J Cancer* **44**: 593–597.

Rothman K, Keller A (1972). The effect of joint exposure to alcohol and tobacco on risk of cancer of the mouth and pharynx. *J Chronic Dis* **25**: 711–716.

Rothman KJ (1976). The estimation of synergy or antagonism. *Am J Epidemiol* **103**: 506–511.

Rothman KJ, Cann CI, Fried MP (1989). Carcinogenicity of dark liquor. *Am J Public Health* **79**: 1516–1520.

Saracci R (1987). The interactions of tobacco smoking and other agents in cancer etiology. *Epidemiol Rev* **9**: 175–193.

Segal I, Reinach SG, deBeer M (1988). Factors associated with oesophageal cancer in Soweto, South Africa. *Br J Cancer* **58**: 681–686.

Talamini R, Franceschi S, Barra S, La Vecchia C (1990). The role of alcohol in oral and pharyngeal cancer in non-smokers and of tobacco in non-drinkers. *Int J Cancer* **46**: 391–393.

Tuyns AJ, Péquignot G, Jensen OM (1977). Le cancer de l'oesophage en Ille-et-Vilaine en fonction des niveaux de consommation d'alcool et de tabac. Des risques qui se multiplient. *Bull Cancer* **64**: 45–60.

Tuyns AJ (1979). Epidemiology of alcohol and cancer. *Cancer Res* **39**: 2840–2843.

Tuyns AJ, Péquignot G, Abbatucci JS (1979). Oesophageal cancer and alcohol consumption; importance of type of beverage. *Int J Cancer* **23**: 443–447.

Tuyns AJ (1983). Oesophageal cancer in non-smoking drinkers and in non-drinking smokers. *Int J Cancer* **32**: 443–444.

Tuyns AJ, Estève J, Raymond L, Berrino F, Benhamou E, Blanchet F, Boffetta P, Crosignani P, Del Moral A, Lehmann W, Merletti F, Péquignot G, Riboli E, Sancho-Garnier H, Terracini B, Zubiri A, Zubiri L (1988). Cancer of the larynx/hypopharynx, tobacco and alcohol: IARC International case-control study in Turin and Varese (Italy), Zaragoza and Navarra (Spain), Geneva (Switzerland) and Calvados (France). *Int J Cancer* **41**: 483–491.

Van Rensburg SJ, Hall JM, Gathercole PS (1986). Inhibition of esophageal carcinogenesis in corn-fed rats by riboflavin, nicotinic acid, selenium, molybdenum, zinc and magnesium. *Nutr Cancer* **8**: 163–170.

Wahrendorf J, Chang-Claude J, Liang QS, Rei YG, Munoz N, Crespi M, Raedsch R, Thurnham D, Correa P (1989). Precursor lesions of oesophageal cancer in young people in a high-risk population in China. *Lancet* **ii**: 1239–1241.

Williams RR, Horm JW (1977). Association of cancer sites with tobacco and alcohol consumption and socioeconomic status of patients: Interview study from the Third National Cancer Survey. *J Natl Cancer Inst* **58:** 525–547.

Wynder EL, Bross IJ, Feldman RM (1957). A study of etiological factors in cancer of the mouth. *Cancer* **10:** 1300–1323.

Wynder EL, Bross IJ (1961). A study of etiological factors in cancer of the esophagus. *Cancer* **14:** 389–413.

Wynder EL, Stellmann SD (1977). Comparative epidemiology of tobacco-related cancers. *Cancer Res* **37:** 4608–4622.

CHAPTER 13

Are Dietary Recommendations in Coronary Heart Disease and Cancer Prevention Compatible?

FJ KOK

Epidemiology Section, TNO Toxicology and Nutrition Institute, Zeist, The Netherlands

The recent dietary recommendations of the National Academy of Sciences are directed to the prevention of chronic disorders, taking into account competing risks for different diseases and nutrient interactions. Among the macro- and micro-components in the diet priority is given to the amount and type of fat.

For coronary heart disease, prominent among the non-malignant disorders, dietary fat is considered most relevant to prevention. For several years, specific goals have been focused on reducing total fat intake to 30% of energy or less, saturated fatty acid intake to less than 10% of energy, and increasing polyunsaturated fatty acid intake to achieve a ratio of near to 1:1 in the intake of saturated and polyunsaturated fatty acids.

Currently the need to lower total fat intake to reduce heart disease risk is questioned. The relevance of high fat consumption in obesity and probably cancer, however, still justifies the recommendation. The main target now is reduction of saturated fat intake to a maximum of 10% of energy. Especially, palmitic acid (16:0), myristic acid (14:0), and lauric acid (12:0) are hyperlipemic and should be reduced, whereas stearic acid (18:0) and short-chain fatty acids are neutral or even beneficial.

A substantial reduction in saturated fat intake requires a replacement source of energy. Although there is uncertainty about the optimal choice, e.g., polyunsaturated fat, monounsaturated fat, and complex or simple carbohydrates, the general advice at present is preferably to increase complex carbohydrate intake. Moreover, vegetable oils containing different types of unsaturated fat may be consumed alternatively. Vegetable oils, however, may be partially hydrogenated during food processing, leading to *trans* unsaturated isomers of oleic acid (18:1) and linoleic acid (18:2), which may exert adverse effects on blood lipids. Since animal experiments suggest increased risk of some cancers, maximising polyunsaturated fat intake is not advocated. In addition, the optimal balance in intake of (n-6) and (n-3) fatty acids, mainly in plant oils and marine fish respectively, is not exactly clear.

From other dietary factors, the protective effect of moderate alcohol consumption and the inverse association with energy intake (probably reflecting beneficial effects of physical activity) are well established. Furthermore, dietary fibre has its contribution, and also antioxidants may turn out to have an impact on preventing coronary heart disease.

In conclusion, opinions are changing on the dietary prevention of coronary heart disease. With the possible exception of alcohol, future recommendations will be better specified and most probably will not conflict with public education on diet and cancer.

PART THREE
MEDITERRANEAN DIET

CHAPTER 14

Mediterranean Diet, Disease and Nutrition Guidelines

A TRICHOPOULOU

Ministry of Health and Welfare, Athens School of Public Health,
Department of Nutrition and Biochemistry, L Alexandras 196,
11521 Athens, Greece

Introduction

Mediterranean diet is a loose term. In Mediterranean countries the local dietary profile rarely corresponds exactly to the purported Mediterranean model, nor is it clear what this model is. It has been common to assume that the Mediterranean diet is a low fat and particularly low saturated fatty acids diet, but there is now evidence that there is more to this diet than just its fatty acid moieties. Thus Greek diet is high in total fat but low in saturated fatty acids whereas the Southern Italian diet is rich in complex carbohydrates and has a low overall fat content. Yet both regions are characterized by very low incidence rates of coronary heart disease (CHD) and several forms of cancers.

Extensive work has been done on the relation of the Mediterranean diet to coronary heart disease, notably by the group of Ancel Keys (1980), but there is also evidence that this diet may contribute, in an as yet undefined way, to the low occurrence of several forms of cancer and other chronic diseases in this region (Berrino and Muti, 1989; Levi *et al.*, 1989).

In this paper I will review the changes taking place in the Mediterranean diet during recent years and will try to assess whether the changes in CHD and cancer occurrence in a number of Mediterranean countries are compatible with the postulated aetiologic links. Four Mediterranean countries were considered: Greece, Italy, Portugal and Spain. These are the four European countries that have traditionally been considered as Mediterranean. Southern France is, of course, as Mediterranean as any other area, but France as a whole is more often thought of as an integral part of the more developed "Western Europe".

The data used were derived mainly from FAO's Food Balance Sheets (Food and Agricultural Organization, 1984) and from WHO's World Health Statistic Annual but other sources were also taken into account.

Table 1 Changes of the average food availability in Greece, Italy, Portugal and Spain, 1961–1985 (in kg per capita per year)

A. Greece

Food groups	1961–65	1971–75	1981–85
Meat	27.0	53.7	68.8
Fish	18.9	14.9	17.6
Milk	129.5	178.4	200.9
Eggs	6.9	10.6	11.3
Cereals	173.2	157.9	143.5
Pulses	8.1	7.1	5.2
Potatoes	33.4	58.0	69.9
Vegetables	104.3	203.2	237.7
Fruits	164.9	170.1	191.8
Sugars	15.9	27.5	34.6
Animal fats			
Vegetable oils	17.3	21.7	24.1
Pure ethanol (lt)	5.3	6.1	6.8

B. Italy

Food groups	1961–65	1971–75	1981–85
Meat	34.6	59.9	76.8
Fish	12.6	12.1	13.9
Milk	154.3	203.5	279.6
Eggs	9.4	11.3	11.6
Cereals	178.5	183.9	161.9
Pulses	5.6	4.4	3.4
Potatoes	48.5	39.8	39.6
Vegetables	132.7	150.3	167.6
Fruits	113.2	131.3	124.1
Sugars	26.4	33.0	30.1
Animal fats	4.1	5.9	8.5
Vegetable oils	14.4	20.3	20.9
Pure ethanol (lt)	13.3	13.4	11.7

Table 1 continued.

C. Portugal

Food groups	1961–65	1971–75	1981–85
Meat	22.1	38.2	45.5
Fish			
Milk	64.6	81.9	98.7
Eggs	3.2	3.6	5.4
Cereals	136.6	136.9	157.6
Pulses	7.0	7.0	5.3
Potatoes	91.6	106.9	96.7
Vegetables	101.4	135.4	132.9
Fruits	78.0	72.5	48.8
Sugars	20.6	27.9	26.7
Animal fats	2.1	2.4	2.8
Vegetable oils	10.1	16.2	16.5
Pure ethanol (lt)	11.1	12.6	18.2

D. Spain

Food groups	1961–65	1971–75	1981–85
Meat	27.2	52.2	70.9
Fish	30.8	37.3	32.2
Milk	92.2	129.9	157.8
Eggs	9.7	13.4	16.3
Cereals	145.8	117.1	114.1
Pulses	7.9	7.6	5.3
Potatoes	112.9	114.2	105.5
Vegetables	136.0	141.5	144.4
Fruits	83.2	121.2	126.0
Sugars	21.6	30.2	30.1
Animal fats	1.7	2.6	2.8
Vegetable oils	15.9	17.3	20.5
Pure ethanol (lt)	9.7	12.0	12.4

Source: Trichopoulou *et al.*, 1990.

Results

Table 1 indicates food availability patterns in the four indicated Mediterranean countries during three 5-year periods spanning a twenty-five-year range (Trichopoulou *et al.*, 1990). There are both geographical and time dependent differences that are partly real and partly reflecting variable

Table 2 Age standarized (World) mortality rates from coronary heart disease and selected cancers, per hundred thousands, by sex, in Greece, Italy, Portugal and Spain (in the early eighties) and their ranks among the corresponding rates of 26 European countries (rank 1 indicates the lowest rate).

		Greece		Italy		Portugal		Spain	
		rate	rank	rate	rank	rate	rank	rate	rank
Ischaemic	M	81.4	4	94.3	5	72.3	2	73.6	3
heart disease	F	30.0	3	38.8	6	32.5	4	29.1	2
Oesophagus	M	1.9	3	4.8	17	5.8	20	5.3	19
cancer	F	0.6	6	0.8	11	1.6	21	0.8	14
Stomach	M	12.1	1	22.7	20	29.7	24	19.8	15
cancer	F	6.7	3	10.7	19	14.5	26	9.8	16
Large bowel	M	7.7	1	18.2	12	16.9	9	11.8	5
cancer	F	6.9	1	13.3	11	12.9	10	9.5	6
Breast cancer	M	—	—	—	—	—	—	—	—
	F	14.6	5	19.2	14	15.0	7	13.5	4
Ovary cancer	M	—	—	—	—	—	—	—	—
	F	2.6	3	4.2	6	2.4	2	2.3	1
Prostate	M	7.3	3	10.8	7	13.8	13	12.8	11
cancer	F	—	—	—	—	—	—	—	—

types of errors in food recording and reporting. There appears to be a decrease in consumption of pulses and, to a lesser extent, cereals and an increase in consumption of eggs, milk products, animal fats and meat. The net results imply a progressive "northernization" of the Mediterranean diet. Further evidence pointing to the same direction comes from Household Budget Surveys (Trichopoulou, 1989) and from *ad hoc* studies in several Mediterranean countries (Ferro Luzzi and Sette, 1989).

Disease occurrence patterns should be based ideally on incidence statistics but such statistics are not available on a country-wide basis in any of the Mediterranean countries. For some diseases, like CHD and most cancer, the high fatality rate allows the use of mortality statistics as substitutes.

Table 2 shows mortality rates, per hundred thousand (age standardized to the world population) for CHD and selected cancers in Greece, Italy, Portugal and Spain, by sex, and their ranks among the corresponding rates of 26 European countries (rank 1 indicates the lowest rate). The cancer sites were chosen as those considered to be more closely related to diet.

Discussion

A comparison among Mediterranean countries or between Mediterranean and other European countries with respect to CHD and cancer mortality rates and food availability patterns may provide some aetiological insights but valid inferences are hindered by unavoidable errors, frequently systematic with respect to both disease reporting and food availability recording. Nevertheless, it is perhaps suggestive that low consumption of animal fats in the Mediterranean countries appears to coincide with the low mortality rates from CHD and cancers of the large bowel, breast, ovary and prostate. By contrast, the expected concordance between high consumption of fruits and vegetables and low mortality from oesophageal and stomach cancer is only evident in Greece and not in the other Mediterranean countries. This may be due to high intake of salty foods or alcoholic beverages in the latter three countries, or to other more subtle methodologic or substantive reasons.

One way to bypass methodological problems built into international correlations is to assess time trends within particular countries of exposures and disease occurrence indicators. In this instance, however, an assumption has to be made about the component cause – specific disease latency.

Figures 1–6 show time trends during the period 1961–85 of the food groups that have been shown or suspected to be related to CHD and the two cancers which are thought of as more strongly related to diet (breast and colorectal). It appears that in the Mediterranean countries the availability of meat, animal fats and vegetable oils is increasing (Figures 1, 2, 3), whereas the availability of cereals and pulses is decreasing, and the availability of vegetables remains stable (with the exception of Greece in which vegetable availability is increasing).

For CHD there is evidence that its occurrence is increasing in the Mediterranean countries, although mortality statistics do not adequately reflect the secular trends because of concommitant treatment improvements. Most of the identifiable dietary changes are compatible with the long-term patterns of CHD occurrence in the indicated Mediterranean countries. For breast cancer there has been little overall improvement in medical treatment during the last 20 years and therefore the mortality trends are interpretable in terms of incidence trends. It appears that increase of either energy intake (which is strongly associated with lipid intake) or of intake of lipids themselves (and particularly animal fat) is associated with an increase of the incidence of breast cancer. These data are not discriminatory as to whether it is fat or energy that is of immediate importance, and do not allow a clear indication as to what is the age at which nutrition is relevant for breast cancer aetiology (perimenarcheal?

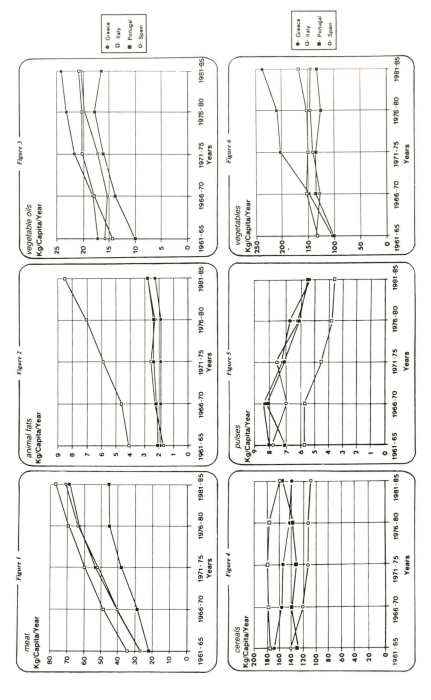

Figure 1 Changes over time of the average daily per capita availability of selected foods in Greece, Italy, Portugal and Spain from 1961 to 1985 (Figures 1–6) (From Trichopoulou, Mossialos, Skalkides. In Hill, Giacosa (eds.) *Causation and Prevention of Human Cancer,* Ch. 3. (Lancaster: Kluwer Academic Publishers)

earlier? later?) but clearly support the notion that nutrition is important in breast cancer causation and that total energy or fat or both are probably implicated.

For colorectal cancer there seems to be an overall increasing trend. The sudden drop between 1977–80 and 1979–80 can only be an artifact, probably attributed to changes in classification practices. The diet link appears likely in view of these data. An increase in meat and fat consumption (vegetable fats may also be hazardous), or the associated increase in energy intake are apparently correlated in time with an increase in the occurrence of colorectal cancer – an increase that cannot be compensated by the modest increase in vegetable intake. Incidentally only in Greece did vegetable intake increase markedly – and only in Greece does colorectal cancer appear to have stabilized during the last few years.

The critical element in the various Mediterranean diets is likely to be their high monounsaturated/saturated ratio (M/S) which is close to or greater than two.

In the existing dietary guidelines it is not mentioned that there are populations with a 40% energy intake from fat which, nevertheless, enjoy good health. The polyunsaturated/saturated ratio is frequently considered in the assessment of a diet without reference to the monounsaturated/saturated and unsaturated/saturated ratios. This may lead to inadequate and possibly misleading evaluation. So, according to most existing guidelines, the Greek population with a 40% energy intake from fat and a relatively low P/S ratio is implicitly advised to change its traditional (and tasteful) way of eating even though this population has one of the longest life expectancies (WHO, 1989); adult Greek males are expected to live longer than their counterparts in USA, UK, Sweden, Denmark, France or Italy, in spite of the notorious Greek smoking habits (Levi *et al.*, 1989).

Conclusion

The data presented here are based on geographical patterns and time trends. Since they are ecological (rather than analytical) they are of limited informativeness. However, this limited information is compatible with existing views concerning the nutritional contribution in the multifactorial aetiology of CHD and at least two common cancers (breast and colorectal). As such, these data strengthen our conviction that nutrition is an important element in overall health policy objectives and that nutrition policy is an important health priority.

Acknowledgement

This study was supported, in part, by a grant from the Greek General Secretariat of Research and Technology (14 YGIONO) to the Athens School of Public Health.

References

Berrino F and Muti P (1989). Mediterranean diet and cancer. In *The Mediterranean Diet and Food Culture* (eds Helsing E, Trichopoulou A); *Eur J Clin Nutr* **43** (Suppl 2): 49–055.

Ferro Luzzi A, Sette S (1989). The Mediterranean diet: an attempt to define its present and past composition. *Eur J Clin Nutr* **43** (Suppl 2): 13–29.

Food and Agricultural Organization. Food Balance Sheets (1984). 1979–1981, Rome.

Food and Agricultural Organization. Personal communicaion.

Levi F, Maisonneuve P, Filiberti R, La Vecchia C, Boyle P (1989). Cancer incidence and mortality in Europe. *Med Soc Prev* **34** (Suppl 2): 51–584.

Keys A (ed) (1980). Seven countries. A multivariate analysis of death and coronary heart diseases. Cambridge, Massachusetts, Harvard University Press.

Trichopoulou A (1989). Nutrition Policy in Greece. *Eur J Clin Nutr* **43** (Suppl 2): 79–82.

Trichopoulou A, Mossialos E, Skalcidis J (1990). Mediterranean diet and cancer. In *Causation and Prevention of Human Cancer* (eds Hill M, Giacosa A); Kluwer, Lancaster.

World Health Organization (1989). World Health Statistics Annual. 158–163.

CHAPTER 15

Mediterranean Diet and Cancer

G VARELA

Department of Nutrition, School of Pharmacy,
Universidad Complutense, Ciudad Universitaria, 28040 Madrid, Spain

The Mediterranean Diet (MeD) may very well serve as an example of the wild oscillations often seen in Science's assessment of some aspect of itself: in just a short time, the MeD has turned, from being held to be rather less than convenient, into its present status of being considered a sort of "catholicon diet". This evidently entails some dangers, as it is obvious that there is no single diet that is "good" for all purposes. Quite the opposite: even in the general information on the diet/health relationship there still remain many doubts and contradictory results. According to Brubacher (1991), this situation is summarized in the following paradox, contained in his prologue to the proceedings of the "Symposium on diet and health in Europe: the evidence": *There remains no doubt about the relationship between diet and health, and yet, in spite of the many studies carried out in recent years, we have no concrete evidence of this relationship.*

For Brubacher, the reasons for this situation are that "on the one hand, the healthy human has very efficient self-regulation systems, and also – often forgotten – the differences in composition and nutritive value of diets show very little effect on health, even though it is true that such effects may accumulate over time. For all these reasons, it is difficult to determine the final effect of a given dietary history on a disease, as the diet is not just an external factor which may affect the disease but also, by itself, a very complex system ("to which we add, and a very difficult one to measure"). This latter problem, that of the measurement of the actual intake, will be the subject of a large proportion of this chapter.

I shall thus try to present to you the opinion of a nutritionist who has spent quite a few years studying the nutrition of Spaniards and the various factors affecting it. Spain is quite rich in alimentary patterns and, even though the mean Spanish diet conforms to the concept of the MeD, marked differences exist between the various Autonomous Communities which constitute Spain, which have also been studied by our group. Furthermore, we have also had the opportunity to cooperate with specialists in various fields of medical pathology in trying to find, in an interdisciplinary approach, some support for the possible relationship between diet and specific diseases or situations: obesity, cardiovascular disease, anorexia nervosa, ageing and, finally, neoplasms of various sites, mainly in the reproductive system.

In trying to relate MeD and cancer, it does seem clear that for certain pathologies, among them some types of cancer, the situation is more favourable in the Mediterranean countries than in those of central and northern Europe. This is attested to by an extensive bibliography (Brubacher, 1991; Keys, 1980; James, 1988; Moreiras-Varela, 1989). On the other hand, if the diets in the Mediterranean countries are different from those in countries further to the north, then it is obvious that the dietetic and non-dietetic risk factors (RF) must also be different, because of the different ecological circumstances and, generally, the different lifestyles of both types of populations. We should in this context remember that, in the Mediterranean countries, these non-dietetic RF's (less stress, "siesta", generally more physical exercise) obviously play an important role (Groot *et al.*, 1991), without however detracting from that of the diet itself. We must also remember that many of these factors, both dietetic and non-dietetic, are convergent, so that the isolated influence of any one of them is very difficult to assess quantitatively.

Furthermore, diet is not a static parameter but one in constant evolution, and in this evolution many other factors intervene. A logical consequence is that knowledge of this evolution over time is of paramount interest, and particularly so in the case of the so-called degenerative diseases, which require a very long implantation period. We should also keep in mind that the MeD has been most intensively studied in its possible relationship to cardiovascular disease, which is where its beneficial aspects first became evident, rather than in its relationship to other conditions, cancer among them.

One of the reasons why knowledge of the diet/health relationship in cardiovascular diseases is much more advanced than that in cancer is that, in the former, it is possible to quantitate the influence of definite dietary factors, most notably the quantity and quality of fats, on cholesterolaemia and the distribution of cholesterol among the various lipoprotein fractions. Regrettably, in the case of cancer, and in spite of the highly valuable insights represented by Wahrendorf's formulas (1987), which try to relate changes in alimentary habits with their role in the possible prevention of some definite neoplasms, we are still very far from the rigour of the Anderson equations (Anderson *et al.*, 1976). These equations allow us to quantify how changes in the energy composition of the diet, and in the energy percentages corresponding to the various families of fatty acids may influence the cholesterolaemia levels.

Keeping these difficulties very much in mind we shall endeavour to find the answers to two questions:

1. Are we today able to deepen our knowledge, with scientific rigour, in the study of the possible diet/cancer relationship?

2. Are the difficulties to be encountered greater when the subject of the study is the Mediterranean diet?

It is, of course, not at all easy to give an answer to these questions, but trying to do so will give us an opportunity to put forward some ideas about the problem. Nevertheless, a few preliminary remarks may be interesting.

Preliminary Remarks

The general problem of the study of the diet/health relationship is logically based, in a first stage (Figure 1) in the background knowledge of the two components of the relation: diet and the relevant condition. With this information, epidemiology in a second stage will strive to find the possible relationship between the two. It is obvious that the lack of reasonable reliability in such information, whether about the diet or about the disease, will render a rigorous scientific study of the relations between the two impossible.

The problem is further complicated by the fact that such a study involves three different types of specialists, all of them working with their own and

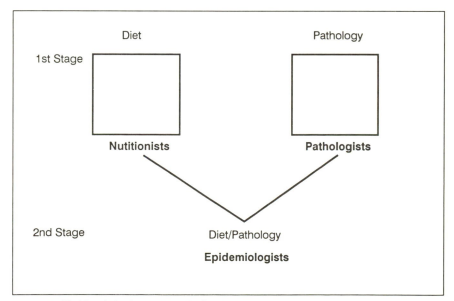

Figure 1 Epidemiologic studies diet/pathology

different methods to arrive at their own and different objectives: dietary intake is the realm of the nutritionist, disease that of the clinician and pathologist, and the relationships between the former and the latter mainly that of the epidemiologist. Not keeping in mind this situation may often lead to mistaken conclusions, as is the case in the subject of this presentation; this stresses the need for cooperation and coordination of methodologies and objectives among the various specialists.

It might be also useful to remember that there is currently a consensus that, in any field of Science (but particularly in those we are discussing), lack of data is preferable to wrong data. There is no need to remind anyone of the disorientations, delays and losses of precious time that have repeatedly arisen because some researcher had absolute faith in data that later turned out to be wrong.

From the point of view of the nutritionist, and in spite of the undoubted complexity of neoplastic disease in its many locations and aetiologies, the information available on cancer morbidity and mortality seems to be more reliable than that on other conditions, such as cardiovascular diseases. Any nutritionist with experience in the study of the nutritional status knows how difficult it is to measure the diet, and in particular its contents in certain given components which might have a relationship to a given disease. A few points may help understand these difficulties.

There is no longer any doubt that, for any biochemical or clinical determination to be valid, it must be accompanied by quality control or validation of the procedure. However, this is often absent in intake measurements, and this may lead to gross errors.

As already pointed out, in any degenerative disease the possibility of the diet behaving as a risk factor will have to be considered not cross-sectionally but longitudinally in time, through the dietary history, and this history should, if possible, extend back to that age at which it is suspected that the influence of the diet in the disease concerned may begin. However, whilst the measurement of the current intake is difficult, retrospective measurements are even more so, in spite of recent important improvements (Varela *et al.*, 1991a). We are thus still quite far from achieving reasonably good reliability in such measurements, and, of course, this reliability is logically always lower than that achieved when studying the current intake. Furthermore, over the period when the diet might influence the development of degenerative diseases changes occur, or may occur, in the quantitative and qualitative composition of that same diet, which are very difficult to assess but should obviously be considered.

A single example may highlight this point: in Spain we have reasonably satisfactory information on the composition of the diet for the country as a whole, for each of the 17 Autonomous Communities and for each of the 50 Provinces, derived from dietary surveys carried out in 1964–65 and in

1980–81 by our own Institute in cooperation with the National Institute of Statistics (Varela *et al.*, 1971, 1985) and from a similar survey carried out by the Ministry of Agriculture, Fishery and Alimentation (1988). Using this database, and after adequate processing, we have recently published (Varela *et al.*, 1991b) a cross-sectional study of the relationship between fat intake – and the various quantitative and qualitative parameters defining it – in the 50 Spanish Provinces and the mortality and morbidity data for the various cancers of the reproductive system for the year 1982.

As would be expected, the results are not satisfactory, for two reasons. Firstly, the changes in the Spanish diet in this period have been quite profound (Varela *et al.*, 1988a; Moreiras-Varela *et al*, 1990). Secondly, the data from the Provinces are means, and it is obvious that, for instance for breast cancer, any correlation should be looked for not for the whole population of the Province but only for the "young female" stratum. This is quite difficult to achieve because of the methodology of the surveys, even if we try, as we have done, to adjust our information to this particular circumstance.

So as to partly obviate these difficulties, we are currently comparing the cancer morbidity and mortality data for the year 1987 with the dietary information derived from the 1964–65 survey. We believe that the time elapsed between both data collection periods might be significant for possible influences on this relationship, and it is our hope that we will thus obtain better information than from a study which is cross-sectional in time.

Difficulties in the Assessment of the Current Diet

It has been noted already that it is not easy to assess the current diet, and even less when the purpose is to look for correlations to a given disease. We have been interested in this subject for a long time, and not only because of possible correlations with cancer. If the methodological approach to the study of the diet/disease relationship is quite different when the disease is due to lack of a given nutrient (deficiency diseases) and when its correlation with nutrition is more complex (as is the case in degenerative diseases) it is quite understandable that the information available about the former is both more extensive and more reliable than about the latter, as deficiency diseases have been until now the most interesting and specialized area of nutritional study. The diagnosis of a deficiency disease generally implies knowing the Recommended Dietary Allowances (RDA) for energy and all nutrients for a given population, and assessing the adequacy of the mean intake of the population.

The problem becomes more complex in the case of degenerative diseases, for a variety of reasons, namely:

(a) Concept of diet.   Confusion sometimes arises regarding this concept which may lead to errors of interpretation of its possible relationship to a given disease. It should be remembered that the human being, in order to be correctly nourished, requires that his diet contain the amount of energy and nutrients needed to fulfil the respective RDAs (Grande and Varela, 1991). These nutrients are normally stored in the foodstuff, but one cannot subsist eating exclusively one single foodstuff because no single foodstuff contains all nutrients in the quantity and quality required to cover the RDAs. Such complete coverage is, however, possible when the diet contains foodstuffs from the various different groups in which they may be classified: fruits, vegetables, cereals, meat, fish, dairy products, etc, as is the case in Spain and in all its Autonomous Communities (Moreira-Varela *et al.*, 1990). This variety in the diet presupposes a correct nutrient density. This means that if the adequate amount of energy is consumed for maintaining a stable weight, this intake will contain all the nutrients required for a balanced diet.

In this area of dietary coverage of the RDAs for energy and the various nutrients in a given population, a confounding factor often arises because the RDAs are estimated on an individual and day basis and according to the age, sex and activity characteristics of the individuals constituting that population. The fact that the RDAs are estimated per day has been taken by some to mean that the intake for each day must be precisely adjusted to the RDAs. This is fortunately not necessary, because for a reasonably well fed and nourished person, the normal situation in the developed countries, generally has sufficient reserves of the various nutrients within his/her body for buffering and compensating day-to-day maladjustments in intake (Varela, 1991).

This stresses the importance of knowing the actual state of such reserves. Generally speaking, in our developed societies it is estimated that it is enough that the diet/RDA adjustment be performed for a period of not less than 15 days. Thus, for instance, a dietary indiscretion (excess or deficiency) over one day has no significance if it is compensated over the other days of this period.

Another consequence is that, from the nutritional point of view and leaving aside the toxicological aspects, there are no "good" or "bad", complete" or "incomplete" foodstuffs. What is to be kept in mind is if the diet is adjusted or not, according to the energy and nutrients supplied, for the coverage of the RDAs over a period of at least 15 days.

(b) Non-nutrient fractions of the diet.   In considering foodstuffs, and therefore diets, besides the nutrient fraction (the only one to interest nutritionists until recently) which contains about 50 nutrients, one must consider a further two non-nutrient fractions (Figure 2). The first one includes the so-called non-nutrient components (NNC); these are natural

Nutritive	No Nutritive	
Energy, nutrients and water No. ≈ 50	Natural compounds No. ?	Additives and contaminants No. ?

Figure 2 Diet composition portions. From G Varela and B Ruiz Roso, 1991

components of the foodstuffs which have been chemically identified; quite a large number of them is known. For instance, the potato, one of the best-studied foodstuffs in this context contains, besides the already mentioned 50 nutrients, over 200 identified components which do not seem to be necessary for human nutrition, and whose role we do not yet know (Varela, 1991). According to Ames, in the mean diet of the developed countries the number of NNC (to which he has given the name of natural additives) is at least 200 times greater than that of the artificial additives intentionally added to the foodstuffs. As shown in the Figure, the second non-nutritional fraction is that formed by additives and contaminants.

Beyond this, however, foodstuffs are generally not consumed raw but only after being subjected to various industrial and culinary processes of conservation, preparation and cooking; it is known that in the course of these processes profound changes in the qualitative and quantitative composition of the nutritional fraction occur (Varela *et al.*, 1990). It is logical to surmise that these changes also affect the non-nutrient fractions, causing not only quantitative changes but also changes in the bio-availability of the components present in the raw foodstuffs. Thus, when we want to relate diet to a given disease we should not only study the possible relationships between the components of the nutrient fraction and the disease, which is what is generally done, but also the possible roles of the other two fractions, certainly not an easy task. The difficulties are due not only to the large number of components in the non-nutrient fractions, but also, for instance, to the new compounds that may arise during the processing of the foodstuffs.

The greatest hurdle in such a study, however, derives from the novelty of the subject itself: the nutritionists' interest was until now focused exclusively on the nutritional fraction, and it is now, when trying to delve deeper into the diet/disease relationship, that we have come to understand the importance of these non-nutritional fractions. This explains the current interest and need to identify these compounds. Until we achieve this goal, a possible first-stage approach to the problem might be that of correlating the various diseases with the individually most important foodstuffs in the diet. Should such a correlation be found, the second stage would be to try to identify the compound or compounds responsible. Yet, information about the presence in a given foodstuff of a compound implicated in this relationship, even if chemically unidentified, would constitute substantial progress.

(c) Regarding methodology. In order to assess the nutritional status of a cohort we need to know the daily intake of nutrients and energy, adjusted to at least 15 days, and to ascertain if this intake is adequate for the coverage of the collective's RDAs. In practice it is necessary that the period of intake measurement last for precisely 15 days; the duration of this period will be governed by the homogeneity of the diet. In general terms, our experience indicates that studying the foodstuffs consumed by a family for seven days is valid for most diets in developed countries, including Spain.

However, this methodology, which is valid for the assessment of the diet's nutrient fraction, might not be valid at all for the non-nutrient fractions.

(d) Substitution effect. Another seemingly trivial fact, which is often disregarded when studying the role of a given foodstuff in the diet in relation to health, is the so-called substitution effect of a foodstuff. When we assess the role of one given foodstuff in the diet, that foodstuff is not consumed in addition to the usual diet, but instead of another one. The substitution of fish for meat, for example, may represent a positive effect as regards cardiovascular diseases. The problem now is to ascertain if this effect is due to eating fish (with its high content of ω-3 fatty acids) or to the fact that one no longer eats meat (rich in saturated fatty acids).

The problem of the diet/cancer relationship is complicated by the discovery, in the NNC fraction of the diet, of various components with marked anti-cancer action (Committee on Diet, Nutrition and Cancer, 1982). For example, vegetables of the genus *Brassica* naturally contain anti-cancer substances which would act by activating dehydrogenases and thus stimulating detoxicating actions on possible carcinogens (Wattenberg, 1977).

Mediterranean Diet and Fat Intake

In a recent paper (Varela and Moreiras, 1991), when discussing the MeD, we pointed out the difficulties in defining it, since it is not uniform among the various countries surrounding the Mediterranean, nor even among the various regions in some of these countries. Furthermore, the traditional diets in these countries are changing markedly, and not always in a positive direction. In spite of these difficulties, however, the dietetic differences

Table 1 **Average fish intake in Spain (Spanish nutritional survey, 1991)**

	PC/day
Total fish	72.0 g
Fatty fish	10.6 g
Sardines	6.6 g

Seasonal changes in the fatty composition of 100 g of sardines

	Total (g)	*SFA* (g)	*MUFA* (g)	*PUFA* $\omega6$	*PUFA* $\omega3$
Summer	20.40	8.49 (41.6%)	6.02 (29.5%)	1.68 (8.2%)	4.22 (20.6%)
Winter	5.4	2.25 (41.6%)	1.23 (22.7%)	0.49 (9.1%)	1.16 (21.4%)

SFA: Saturated fatty acids.
MUFA: Monounsaturated fatty acids.
PUFA: Polyunsaturated fatty acids.
(Varela and Ruiz-Roso, 1989)

between these countries and those of central and northern Europe seem clear. Further, it seems to be equally clear that these dietetic differences are somehow associated with differences in mortality and morbidity, particularly for cardiovascular diseases and possibly also some cancers. Among the various components of the MeD, fat is the one receiving the most interest in this context.

Estimation of fat intake is generally difficult, particularly in the case of the MeD. For example, the beneficial effects of food consumption in cardiovascular diseases are known and are mainly due to its polyunsaturated ω-3 fatty acids. However, it is not enough to speak about overall consumption of fish. As observed in our laboratory (Table 1), there are marked seasonal variations, both quantitative and in the composition of the various fatty acid families, and these variations may logically influence the fat/health relationship.

Nevertheless, the greatest difficulty in the assessment of the true lipid intake derives from other sources. Most of the information on the dietary fat/health relationship stems from experimental or epidemiological studies in which the fat intake is calculated from the foodstuffs consumed, with the help of Food Composition Tables. However, in most of these tables the fat content and composition given is that in the raw foodstuffs, while most of these are consumed after being subjected to various industrial and – most importantly – home or institutional cooking processes. In the course of these procedures, the fat composition of the foodstuffs undergoes important quantitative and qualitative changes, which obviously modify the composition of the lipid intake (Varela *et al.*, 1990; Varela, 1988; Varela

Table 2 Differential characteristics of the Mediterranean diet fat intake

1. Composition

	Quantitative composition:	≈
	Qualitative composition	Dietetic cholesterol ↓
		SFA ↓↓
		MUFA ↑↑
		PUFA ω6 ↑
		PUFA ω3 ↑

2. Intake

    a.   Low butter and margarine intakes
    b.   High vegetable oils intake, mainly olive oil
    c.   50% of the total fat intake is culinary fat
    d.   Most of the culinary fat is used in deep-frying

Note:
↑ means high consumption in Mediterranean diet.
↓ means lower consumption in Mediterranean diet.
Double arrow represents quantitative differences.
Varela, 1991.

et al., 1988b). The differential features of the fat intake in the MeD, (Table 2) depend not only on its food composition, but also on the form in which those food are consumed. One of the characteristics of the MeD is that about 50% of the total fat intake is not derived from the foodstuffs themselves, but from the cooking fats with which they are prepared which has evident advantages from the nutritional point of view. This immediately begs the question, "how is this cooking fat consumed?". Basically, only a small fraction of this cooking fat is consumed raw, in dressings; most of it is used for frying foods. Our interest was first directed at the study of the deep-frying (DF) process. The progress achieved in the knowledge of the penetration of fat into the foods has possibly transformed ideas about this technique. Previously considered less than convenient in non-Mediterranean countries, it is today one of the most widespread cooking techniques in countries and for foodstuffs where it was previously unpopular. Building on the data of fat penetration during deep-frying, we then turned to other procedures, both home-cooking (stir-frying, stewing) and industrial (canning), where various different types of cooking fats are used (Varela *et al.*, 1988b; Perez Alvarez-Quiñones, 1990; Varela, 1990).

The process of DF foodstuffs is a highly complex one (Varela *et al*, 1988b), in which many factors have a role. These factors may be broadly classified into three categories: (a) those depending on the process itself, (b) those depending on the type of cooking fat, and (c) those depending on the foodstuff. Such is the complexity of this process that, for some authors (Dagerskog, 1977), "frying is the most important and difficult

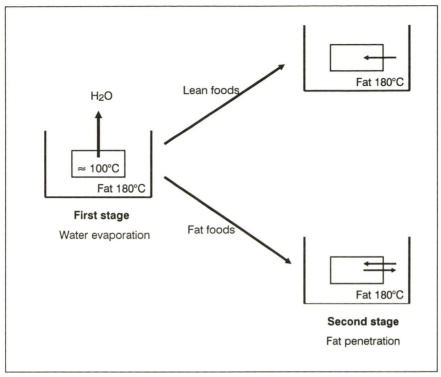

Figure 3 Fat penetration in foods in deep frying. (From G Varela and B Ruiz-Roso, 1991)

operation in the industrial or institutional preparation of food". In principle DF essentially consists in replacing part of the water contained in the foodstuff with the cooking (frying) fat which penetrates into it. For this penetration of the hot fat (at about 180°C) to occur, most of the water must first evaporate, and in potatoes during this phase, the core temperature within the foodstuff remains at about 100°C (Varela *et al.*, 1988b) (Figure 3). When the process is correctly carried out as the fat penetrates into the foodstuff it builds a sort of peripheral crust which prevents its deeper penetration into the mass of the foodstuff. Olive oil (OO) has shown itself to be particularly adequate for this form of frying.

Some practical consequences of this form of frying are:

(a)   The action time of the hot fat on the interior of the foodstuffs is really very short, and in the absence of oxygen. The outcome of these two factors is that DF is a less aggressive process to the heat-labile components of the foodstuff than other cooking procedures. For instance, the loss of vitamin C in various vegetable foodstuffs is much smaller in DF than in other cooking processes.

Table 3 Changes in fat composition due to frying

	LEAN FOOD		FAT FOOD		
	Potatoes		Sardines		
	Raw	Fried OO	Raw	Fried OO	Fried SFO
Total fat	0.16	16.5*	20.2	20.3	20.2
SFA	23.1	12.2	42.4	30.6*	26.4*
MUFA	3.1	78.2*	29.5	46.0*	32.8
PUFA (Total)	73.1	8.4*	26.6	23.1	33.6*
ω6			4.9	6.6	26.2*
ω3			21.3	16.5	7.0*

Total fat expressed as g/100 g of food and fatty acids families in g/100 g of fat.
OO   = Olive oil
SFO = Sunflower oil
* = Significant as opposed to raw ($p < 0.05$)
Varela and Ruiz-Roso, 1991.

Table 4 Changes in the lipidic composition of lean and fat, raw and fried in olive oil, beef meat

	Beef meat				
	OO	LEAN		FAT	
	Raw	Raw	1st frying	Raw	1st frying
Total fat (g/100 g food)	100	3.1	6.4*	41.0	40.8
SFA	15.7	41.2	28.6*	43.8	42.0*
MUFA	74.4	43.2	61.5*	49.5	52.0*
PUFA (g/100 g total fat)	9.7	15.6	9.6*	2.3	2.0

Total fat expressed as g/100 g of food and fatty acids families in g/100 g of fat
OO   = Olive oil
*   = Significant as opposed to raw ($p < 0.05$)
Varela and Ruiz-Roso, 1991.

(b)   The replacement of water by fat and the formation of the surface crust markedly increase the palatability of the fried foodstuffs, rendering them more acceptable for man.

(c)   Because of the peculiar penetration kinetics, and when the procedure is correctly carried out, the amount of fat ingested with the fried foodstuffs is not greater than with other cooking procedures.

(d)   During the DF process important qualitative changes occur in the fat composition of the foodstuff, so that the true lipid intake with the fried foodstuff is quite different from its raw composition.

The fat penetration into foods varies between lean and fatty foodstuffs (Figure 3). In both cases, it is necessary that in a first phase, prior to the penetration of the fat, a sizable amount of water be expelled from the foodstuff through evaporation. During this phase the inner temperature of the foodstuff remains practically constant at 100°C. Once the water has evaporated fat penetration into the foodstuff begins. For lean foods, the fat in the frying bath will penetrate into the foodstuff, which will therefore become enriched in fat; logically, the composition of the fried foodstuff will be practically the same as that of the original cooking fat. Where fatty foodstuffs are concerned, the quantity of fat passing from the deep-frying bath to the foodstuff, and *vice versa*, is about the same. Thus, there are no significant changes in the quantity of fat in the fried foodstuff as compared with the raw one. There are however differences from the qualitative point of view and these will largely depend on the concentration gradients of the various fatty acids between the cooking fat and the foodstuff itself. Generally, there is a trend for both concentrations to become equal, and this implies a change in the fatty acid composition, both in the cooking fat (which will be enriched in those fatty acids which pass into it from the foodstuff) and conversely in the foodstuff, which will become enriched in those fatty acids penetrating into it from the cooking (frying) fat. Table 3 shows, as an example, the changes observed when frying potatoes (lean foods) and sardines (fatty foods) in olive oil (Perez Alvarez-Quiñones, 1990), which has a very high content of oleic acid (MUFA). In the first case, as was to be expected, the lipid composition of the fried foodstuff is very rich in MUFA, derived from the olive oil in the frying bath. In the second, the total lipid content of the sardines is practically unchanged.

A further example is the changes in lipid composition when frying lean or fatty meat in olive oil. For lean meat, the total lipid content increases with a marked decrease of the SFA fraction while the MUFA increase and the PUFA decrease (Table 4). When fatty meat is fried the quantitative changes are non-significant, as the amount of fat lost into the bath and that penetrating from the bath are practically the same. As expected the proportion of SFA decreases, the MUFA increase, and there are no

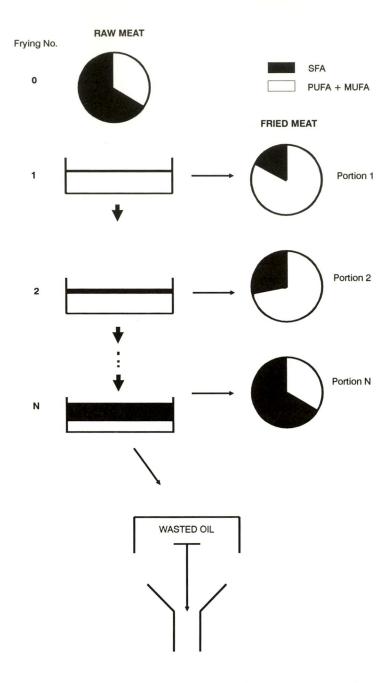

Figure 4 Quantity and quality of the fat intake in repeated meat frying (From G Varela *et al.*, 1990)

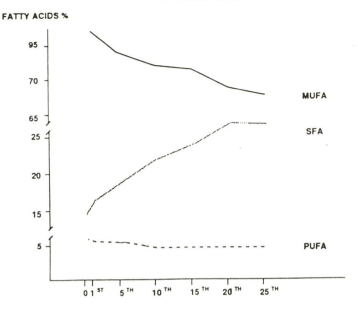

Figure 5 Changes in fatty acid composition in repeated fryings of fat meat in olive oil (From G Varela and B Ruiz-Roso, 1991)

variation in the PUFA fraction, as the concentrations of this family in the meat used and in the oil are very similar.

The effects of the fat are not the same when ingested alone as they are when ingested in the fried foodstuff. When frying foodstuffs, the same oil is used several times for frying new portions of the foodstuff. This aspect of repeated frying (RF) is quite important, and closely related to the so-called "useful life" of cooking fats (Varela *et al.*, 1983). How many times those fats may be used in such RF is very difficult to assess, as it will depend on many factors, and particularly on the lipid composition of the raw foodstuff and the type of cooking oil concerned. In this context, it is well known that olive oil, because of its composition (high MUFA and low PUFA content) is much more stable than other PUFA-rich oils.

In RF, a moment arrives when the oil used in RF is no longer usable and must be discarded (Figure 4). The amount of this discarded oil may be considerable, depending (among other factors) on the lipid composition of the cooking fat and the foodstuff and on the stability of the cooking fat itself, so it may be of practical importance for the actual lipid intake. It is not easy to estimate the amount of oil discarded, but it must exceed 25% of the original "raw" amount, as this is the proportion of polar compounds generated during frying that marks the cut-off point from which the oil must be discarded (Dobarganes and Perez-Camino, 1985). However, this discarded oil does not have the same composition as the original "raw" one, but has been enriched in saturated fatty acids (Figure 5). In practical terms, this means that we have on the one hand reduced the total lipid intake, and on the other eliminated negative compounds (and not only for cardiovascular disease) such as SFA. Furthermore, the lipid composition of the meat is substantially improved because of the fatty acids it acquires, such as ω-3 or ω-6 PUFA depending on the cooking oils used.

It should be stressed that when a heat-stable oil such as olive oil is used for frying meat, the number of RF that can be carried out is much greater than for other foodstuffs, for instance fish. The high PUFA content in fish, part of which passes into the oil and reduces its heat stability, restricts the number of repeated fryings that may be carried out.

Even in RF the meat loses SFA and is enriched in MUFA; this is highly positive for its possible correlation with various diseases, among them cardiovascular diseases; together with the discarded oil we eliminate from the diet a proportion of these SFA. The experiments described here have been performed in domestic fryers where the cooking fat/foodstuff volume ratio is large, so that the observed changes in oil composition are much slower than would be observed, if a frying pan had been used (where the volume ratio is much lower).

Finally, we have also studied the fat penetration patterns into foodstuffs when using other cooking techniques or industrial processes, such as canning fish in various types of oil. The results observed have been in the same general direction, though not of the same magnitude (Perez Alvarez-Quiñones, 1990; Varela, 1990).

Conclusion

We have tried to present and discuss some of the difficulties encountered in the assessment of true intake, which is the required basis for establishing scientifically rigorous correlations with different diseases and therefore with cancer. These difficulties increase when we try to study lipid intake, which is one of the differentiating features of the Mediterranean diet.

We believe it is important to identify these difficulties so that, working together, we may be able to solve them and thus progress in the knowledge of the interrelationships between diet and cancer.

References

Anderson JT, Grande F, Keys A (1976). Independence of the effects of cholesterol in man. *Am J Clin Nutr* **28**: 1184.

Brubacher GB (1991). Preface Diet and Health in Europe: the evidence. *Ann Nutr Metab* **35** (Suppl 1):

Committee on Diet, Nutrition and Cancer (1982). National Research Council, National Academy Press, Washington DC.

Dagerskog M (1977). Time-temperature relationships in industrial cooking and frying. In *Physical Chemical Changes in Food Caused by Thermal Processing* (eds Hoyem T, Kvale O); Appl Sciences Publ, London.

de Groot L, van Stavaren W, Hautvast JGAJ (1991). Nutrition and the elderly in Europe. EURONUT-SENECA (CEE). *Eur J Clin Nutr* **45** (Suppl 3):

Dobarganes MG, Perez-Camino MC (1985). Métodos analiticos de aplicación en grasas calentadas. I. Determinación de esteres metilicos de dimeros no polares. *Grasas y Aceites* **35**: 351–7.

Grande F, Varela G (1991). En busca de la Dieta Ideal. Publicaciones de la Fundación Española de la Nutrición. Serie Divulgación No 12, Madrid.

James WPT (1988). *Healthy Nutrition. Preventing nutrition-related diseases in Europe*. WHO. Regional Office for Europe European Series No 24. Copenhagen.

Keys A (1980). *Seven Countries. A multivariate study of death and coronary heart diseases*. Cambridge (USA), Harvard University Press.

Ministerio de Agricultura, Pesca Y Alimentacion. Consumo alimentario en España (1987). Publicaciones de la Dirección General de Politica Alimentaria, Madrid.

Moreiras-Varela O (1989). The Mediterranean diet in Spain. *Eur J Clin Nutr* **43** (Suppl 2): 83–7.

Moreiras-Varela O, Perez I, Carbajal A (1990). Evolución de los hábitos alimentarios en España. Publicaciones del Ministerio de Sanidad y Consumo, Madrid.

Perez Alvarez-Quiñones M (1990). El proceso de enlatado de sardinas. Repercusiones nutricionales y sensoriales de la fritura y de las diferentes fases de elaboración y maduración. Tesis Doctoral. Facultad Farmacia, Universidad Complutense, Madrid.

Varela G, Garcia D, Moreiras-Varela O (1971). La Nutrición de los españoles. Diagnóstico y Recomendaciones. Publicaciones del Instituto de Desarrollo Económico, Madrid.

Varela G, Moreiras-Varela O, Ruiz-Roso B (1983). Utilización de algunos aceites en frituras repetidas. Cambios en las grasas y análisis sensorial de los alimentos fritos. *Grasas y Aceites* **34**: 101–7.

Varela G, Moreiras-Varela O, Requejo A (1985). Estudios sobre Nutricion (2 Volumenes). Publicaciones del Instituto Nacional de Estadistica, Madrid.

Varela G (1988). Role de l'huile d'olive dans la preparation des aliments. *Rev Franc Corp Grass* **35**: 215–222.

Varela G, Moreiras O, Carbajal A (1988a). Evolución del estado nutritivo y de los hábitos alimentarios de la población española. Publicaciones de la Fundación Española de la Nutrición. Seri Divulgación No. 9, Madrid.

Varela G, Bender AE, Morton ID (1988b). Frying of food. Principle changes, new approaches. Ellis Horwood, Chichester, UK.

Varela G (1990). Changes in fat composition due to industrial and culinary processing. Possible consequences in prevention of cardiovascular diseases. 4th International Colloquium on Mono-unsaturated fatty acids. Congress on the biological value of olive oil. Boston, USA.

Varela G, Perez M, Ruiz-Roso B (1990). Changes in the quantitative and qualitative composition of fat from fish, due to seasonality and industrial and culinary processing. *Bibl Nutr Dieta* **46:** 104–9.

Varela G (1991). Dietay Salud. *Rev Sanidad e Higiene Pública* **65:** 77–81.

Varela G, Moreiras O (1991). Mediterranean diet. *Cardiovascular Risk Factors* **1:** 313–321.

Varela G, Moreiras O, Carbajal A, Belmonte S (1991a). Estudio transversal entre la cantidad y calidad de la grasa consumida en España y la mortalidad por diferentes tipos de neoplasias del aparato reproductor. *Rev Clin Española* **189:** 55–9.

Varela G, Moreiras O, Carbajal A, Belmonte S (1991b). Estudio de la relación entre la grasa de la dieta y el cáncer de mama en España. Informe a la Fundación Banco Exterior, Madrid.

Wahrendorf J (1987). An estimate of the proportion of colo-rectal and stomach cancer which may be prevented by certain changes in dietary habits. *Int J Cancer* **40:** 625–8.

Wattenberg LW (1977). Naturally occurring inhibitors of chemical carcinogenesis. In *Naturally Occurring Carcinogens-Mutagens and Modulators of Carcinogenesis*; (ed Miller), Jap Soc Scien Press, Tokyo, pp. 315–29.

PART FOUR
CONSIDERATIONS WHEN
GIVING ADVICE

CHAPTER 16

Ethics of Dietary Advice for Cancer Prevention

A GIACOSA[1], P VISCONTI[1], R FILIBERTI[2], F MERLO[2]

[1]Nutritional Unit, [2]Epidemiology Unit
National Institute for Cancer Research, Genova, Italy

With the conquest of most infectious diseases, cancer and heart disease have emerged as the two major causes of death in the western world. Although progress has been made in the treatment of some cancers (e.g. leukaemias, testicular cancer, endometrial cancer) and in early detection (e.g. cervical cancer) the most likely way to decrease the mortality from cancer is prevention. To do this we need to know the cause of the cancer, the best way to remove the cause, and any possible side-effects of removal of the cause, so that a cost-benefit analysis can be made (Hill, 1988).

Doll and Peto (1981) estimated that approximately 35% of all cancers are due to smoking. Much smaller percentages are caused by radiation, chemical exposure, viruses etc. The proportion of cancer mortality which may be attributable to dietary factors, at least in the USA, has been estimated by the same authors at 35%, though with a wide margin of uncertainty from 10% to 70% (Doll and Peto, 1981). The equivalent proportion of cancer incidence due to diet has been estimated at about 40% and 60% for males and females, respectively by Wynder and Gori (1977), while Higginson and Muir (1979) gave estimates of 30% and 63% for Birmingham, UK and 18% and 58% for Bombay, India. Dietary influences on cancer risk were estimated by these authors to be at least as important as tobacco exposure, yet the role of diet in the causation of cancer has been difficult to study, partly because "diet" encompasses such a wide variety of foods and dietary habits, but also because the means by which these habits can be measured are difficult to apply to large numbers of individuals. These difficulties are reflected in the uncertainty surrounding the overall risk of cancer that is attributable to what we eat. When we look at individual cancer sites, although there are some areas of certainty, in most cases we need more information. According to Hill (1988) the causes can be divided as:

(a)   Areas of certainty:
      Smoking: lung; bladder; pancreas.

(b)   Areas where the information is good:
      Obesity: endometrium; breast.
      Promiscuity: cervix.

(c)   Areas where the information is weak:
      dietary fat/fibre/calories: colon; breast; stomach; oesophagus.

Despite the difficulties in interpreting the evidence on diet and cancer, several agencies have issued dietary guidelines intended to reduce cancer risk.

For most of the common cancers, except lung cancer, (e.g. breast, colon, stomach, pancreas) there is good evidence that diet is important, but the evidence concerning which dietary items is weak. This creates two major ethical problems.

The first of these is whether we are allowed to issue dietary guidelines for the general public in order to reduce cancer incidence. If the answer here is yes, then the second problem is whether we go further and try to persuade people to change their diet. In order to try to clarify these problems the following topics will be addressed:

1.   What is health?

2.   What is the role of ethics in nutritional advice?

3.   Health education and health promotion: how do they relate to the rights of the individual:

4.   Is it better to talk about nutrition and cancer prevention or prevention of nutrition-related diseases?

What is Health?

The literature of health education tends nowadays to take a complex view of the concept of health and to distinguish various elements within it and particularly to differentiate between "negative" and "positive" health. The concept of "negative health", is associated with the absence of ill-health. "Ill-health" itself is a complex notion comprising disease, illness, handicap, injury, and other related ideas (Downie, 1990). These overlapping concepts can be linked if they are seen on the model of abnormal, unwanted or incapacitating states of a biological system (Downie *et al.*, 1990; Seedhouse, 1986).

The concept of "positive health" has more recently appeared in published reports. The origins of this idea are in the definition of health to be found in the preamble to the Constitution of the World Health Organization (WHO): "Health is a state of complete physical, mental and social well-being, and not merely the absence of disease or infirmity" (WHO, 1946). It follows from this definition that "well-being" is an important ingredient in positive health.

A third idea in the concept of health is that of "fitness". Fitness is a term that is often used by the general public to describe the state of someone's heart and lungs function, or the ability to achieve a set of physical activities without any difficulty. But fitness can also be used in a related but broader sense, which Downie calls the "sociological" as opposed to the "heart and lungs" sense (Downie, 1990). In the sociological sense of fitness a person is fit for some occupation or job. This means that people have the necessary health to enable them to perform the job or task adequately without, for example, too many days off work.

The fact that health (the absence of ill-health) and well-being cannot be measured on a linear scale must raise the question of whether they are in fact two components of a single concept. According to Downie *et al.* (1990) the conclusion could be that while the concepts of health and well-being overlap, they are distinct entities and cannot be combined into one concept (Downie *et al.*, 1990).

What is "Ethics" in Medicine?

Medical associations or policy makers are trying to define new codes of ethics. In an essay by David Roy and Maurice AM de Wachter in "Traité d' Anthropologie médicale", the point is made that any new deontology will have to emerge from within the rationale of the biomedical sciences and the practice of medicine (Roy and de Wachter, 1988). "Nous sommes sur le point de reconnaitre que la déontologie médicale est une question de jugement clinique, et non pas seulement une spécialisation de la réflexion philosphique, ou une intrusion des humanités en médecine". (We are on the point of recognizing that medical deontology is a question of clinical judgement, and not only a branch of philosophy, or an intrusion of the humanities into medicine).

What, then, is the key to an ethic of proper lifestyle? In a general and ill-defined way, the new concept that seems to be gaining momentum in public opinion is the one of "quality of life". The phrase is now invested with an undefined, general meaning applicable to both collective and individual behaviour. It may be used with reference to malformed fetuses or euthanasia, as well as to procedures surrounding terminal cancers (e.g. palliative care units). Bégin (1988) calls it a new shared value, possibly the basis of a common ethic of which the elements are still unravelled.

Obviously the concept is even more important if it can also be introduced when promoting healthy lifestyles (Bégin, 1988).

In this regard two difficulties must be recognized. The first is that lifestyles are very resistant to change. This resistance is caused by cultural tradition and by its geographical variability. Even within nations and local cultures the variation in eating and drinking habits is considerable. With this background it is obvious that health education should represent a balance between ethnic and social tolerance on one side, and the need for active prevention on the other. In the opinion of Riis' (1990) the mere act of collecting scientific data on eating and drinking habits can lead to an ethically significant risk of stigmatizing certain groups.

The second difficulty is related to the need to recognize people's fear of spending their life acting as if they are ill subjects simply in order to die healthy. The magnitude of the necessary safeguards needed to live "healthily" may exceed the magnitude of the perceived risk. For example, where people perceive heart disease to be sudden death they may regard it as inconvenient rather than something to fear. If, in contrast, they regard it as the risk of spending their last years in a state of helpless incapacity, this would provoke more fear and make drastic changes in lifestyle seem more acceptable. Consequently the ethical implications in nutritional policy making have to be properly defined and in particular the relationships between individual freedom and health promotion has to be clarified. This could be included in the domain of behavioural ethics!

Health Education

At a very general level health education is "an activity aimed at restoring, maintaining, or enhancing the health of individuals and communities".

In Downie's opinion this statement is not adequate for it provides at best a necessary and not a sufficient definition of health education (Downie, 1990). Moreover, according to this author, the definition as stated could apply to the work of doctors but not to the work of health educators in general. Medicine typically stresses the curative or palliative, whereas health education stresses the preventive. In addition, it could be said that medicine stresses the doctor-patient or one-to-one relationship, whereas health education tends to have a broader societal perspective (Downie, 1990). Downie considers also that medicine tends to be reductivist in its assumptions (following from the scientific study of disease processes on which it is based) whereas health education tends to be holistic in its assumptions (Downie, 1990).

From these distinctions, it follows that health education gives rise to an acute set of moral problems because it is interfering with lifestyle in general rather than in the individual. It therefore requires considerable ethical justification.

Health Promotion

When discussing health, it is fundamentally important to distinguish between health education and health promotion. It might be said that traditionally health education has been concerned with negative health, whereas health promotion is concerned with positive health, but this does not appear correct (Doxiadis, 1987).

A second superficial contrast is that health education, like all true education, would respect the autonomy of its recipients, whereas health promotion bypasses autonomy and sells health "like a commodity"; in its extreme forms it can resemble the advertisements for unhealthy products which it is opposing (Williams, 1984).

In reply to this argument it could be questioned whether all true education actually does respect autonomy. It might be maintained that autonomy is not something which everyone in fact possesses. People can be victims of all sorts of social processes and be lacking in power. Downie (1990) says that is quite unrealistic to regard all recipients of health education as autonomous. The author underlines that education of any kind, whether concerned with health or not, must take into account the fact that people, young or old, must be "empowered", and education is an important part of the process of empowerment. It must aim at creating or enhancing autonomy, but should not presuppose it. This issue is ethically important and should be examined in more detail. Is health education really "education" or is it rather "training", "instruction", or even "indoctrination"? Downie *et al.* (1990) define health education as an activity aimed at preventing ill-health and furthering positive health, through creating an understanding of the human body and its workings, through the provision of information about health services and access to them, and through creating understanding of national or local policies and environmental processes which may be detrimental to health.

It follows from this definition that health education is indeed education in the fullest sense. But it also follows that health education cannot be widely effective on its own but needs to be supplemented by, and seen in the wider perspective of, health promotion if it is to be effective. This approach to health education and health promotion is in agreement with the policy of WHO (1984).

Downie (1990) summarizes the relationship between health education, health promotion, and prevention as shown in Figure 1.

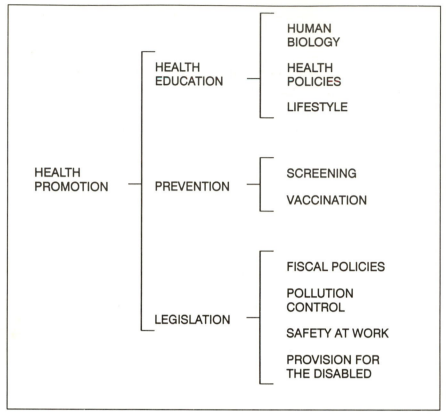

Figure 1 Relationship between health education, health promotion and prevention

Dietary Guidelines

Coming back to the basic topic of this chapter we will discuss now the ethical implications of dietary guidelines. Several organizations in different countries have issued dietary guidelines for the public in order to reduce cancer incidence. Meanwhile, proponents and opponents of dietary guidelines disagree about their justification. The two main arguments which result in people becoming either proponents or opponents are the judgement on scientific evidence and the process of decision making.

Surely, the need for reliable information in health education represents a place where ethics and science meet prevention. But, as previously described, the evaluation of all scientific evidence on the diet-cancer issue suggests various problems (de Vet and van Leeuwen, 1986); principally:

1.   No criteria are available for taking into account the methodological weaknesses of each individual study.

2.   No criteria are available for determining the weight that should be given to different types of studies.

3.   There is disagreement concerning how much needs to be known about the adverse effects of a specific recommendation on other cancers and other diseases.

4.   There is no consensus about the question of whether intervention studies should be performed before recommendations can be discussed.

The second problem in making dietary recommendations is the process of decision making. This point however implies that in addition to health-related aspects, other arguments, such as economical, sociological, psychological, ethical, philosophical and education aspects, also play a role in the decision about dietary guidelines (de Vet and van Leeuwen, 1986).

In particular the ethical implications have to be underlined. De Vet and van Leeuwen (1986) think that with ethical aspects, the very essentials of making recommendations to the public are at stake. This is because health professionals, by proposing recommendations, impose a health norm on the population and presume that they know what is best for all of us. Thus, health education becomes health propaganda (aimed directly at behavioural change) and is no longer based on informed individual decisions about health behaviour (Miettinen, 1983).

They regard this as an unfortunate development because individuals have widely divergent views on the extent to which they are willing to sacrifice life's amenities for their health. They believe that individuals themselves should weigh the health-related aspects of recommendations together with other factors. As a consequence, the population needs more information on the diet-cancer issue than it presently receives.

Proponents of guidelines usually argue that recommendations are not orders and that individuals can freely choose whether or not to conform to them. This may be true in theory, but in practice it is evident that the public receives guidelines as authoritative rules for good health (de Vet and van Leeuwen, 1986). This misconception can only be altered by promoting health education of a less "normative" nature.

Proponents of guidelines sometimes argue that it is unethical to withhold recommendations from the public. In this regard, the National Research Council of USA (1982) stated: "......the consequences of failure to act are so important that we should proceed at once to try to alter people's diet in an attempt to reduce the risk of cancer". In support of this statement, many authors pointed out that more timely campaigns against smoking would have prevented many tobacco-related cancer deaths: thus probably we could compare the status of diet-cancer evidence now to that of smoking and lung cancer about 20 years ago. However, in this situation we have to be careful because it may appear illogical and erroneous to compare different problems, different times and different levels of knowledge.

In summary, it can be concluded that it is certainly unethical to withhold knowledge from the public, but equally it is unethical to make recommendations that imply promises that cannot be supported with strong evidence.

What to Do?

We lack scientific answers to a large number of fundamental questions dealing with food and drink, but this fact should not paralyse us. To wait for more reliable scientific information on those topics, and many others, could lead to a kind of defeatism in which any initiative could be postponed because "we still do not know enough". The ideal should be to transform reliable research results into active intervention through health education in a constantly progressing way. But if we look at past experience, we realise that other aspects have to be considered.

If we analyse the changes in recent years that have led towards better lifestyles, we observe the following (Bégin, 1988):

–   Combat of over-eating and lack of exercise: these changes were promoted by the private sector, who sold an idealized body shape to consumers on the basis of the notion of social achievement and on images of the good life.

–   Combat of smoking: changes have been achieved through the development of a new consensus in society.

–   Combat of dangerous driving: changes were achieved initially by legislation, apparently ahead of public opinion, but then accepted by the majority.

–   Combat of abuse of pharmaceuticals: here changes are taking place through the intervention of various associations and through the increase of costs (at least in some countries, i.e. Italy).

However no positive changes were seen on other fronts, particularly in diet. On the contrary, large and potentially negative modifications were seen in diet habits in the last 30 years, with the adoption of the so-called "Western diet" (high calorie, high fat, low fibre diet) in most European countries and the progressive abandonment of traditional models in Mediterranean areas.

Most of these modification were promoted by publicity from the food producers and by social changes which followed the Second World War. It is well known that social change is rarely the linear, rational, path one dreams of developing, nor does it follow the prescriptions of policy documents. Under these circumstances is it really unethical to produce diet guidelines for the general population?

The Prevention of Nutrition-Related Diseases of Major Public Health Importance

It is apparent from many literature reports that a common set of dietary recommendations is suggested for the prevention of many diseases of major public health importance, including cancer (US Nat Res Council, 1982).

For example, the evidence for the role of diet in the development of cardiovascular disease points to the need to limit saturated fatty acid intake. This, in many countries, is most readily achieved by limiting total fat intake. The recommendations for the prevention of obesity include the suggestion that the total fat and sucrose content of the diet should fall. These two recommendations aim to reduce the energy density and increase the nutrient density of the diet. Both children and adults will need to adjust their intakes by eating increased amounts of starchy food to cover their energy needs. The resulting effects on the general nutritional state are likely to be beneficial because mineral and vitamin intakes are likely to rise, thus minimizing other nutritional problems such as iron deficiency anaemia.

An increase in cereal, root vegetable and fruit consumption must form the main part of the compensatory response to the decline in fat and sugar intakes. This would also meet the recommendation that dietary fibre intakes should increase in order to prevent constipation and diverticula disease. Dietary potassium would also rise. These changes are likely to be particularly beneficial in the elderly, and in other groups where the total energy intake is low. A common pattern of changes in food consumption emerges from these recommendations and it is possible to produce a coherent plan for the prevention of several diseases. It is not necessary to argue for dietary change on the basis of only one dietary effect: a fall in sucrose intake, for example, is beneficial for several reasons in addition to the prevention of dental caries. It is also not necessary to propose only one way of compensating for the reduction in fat and sugar intake. The type of cereals, fruit or vegetables – or low fat milk, meat or fish products – will obviously depend on the prevailing national food habits and the availability of alternative products.

The proposed changes in diet in many European countries can be achieved provided manufacturing practices alter to allow the provision of foods with a higher nutritional value. For example it will be shown that salt intakes depend particularly on the addition of salt to products by food manufacturers. If cereal consumption is to rise then the high salt content of bread and breakfast cereals will need to fall appreciably to allow both an increase in cereal consumption and a fall in salt intakes.

All these indications (mostly coming from the WHO analysis and planning) prove that it is possible nowadays to plan dietary guidelines that are contemporaneously useful for the prevention of cardiovascular diseases and other pathological conditions of major social interest (i.e. dental caries, diabetes, constipation, diverticulosis, overweight, etc) and at the same time are helpful in preventing cancer (Nat Res Council, 1982).

Conclusions

Interaction of ethics, health policy, nutritional guidelines and cancer prevention still contain uncertainties and debatable aspects. But a balanced analysis of the assumptions previously discussed, clearly could justify – from the ethical point of view – the diffusion in the general population of dietary guidelines for cancer prevention, given that they can be considered properly relevant for the prevention of many diseases other than cancer itself.

References

Bégin M (1988). Lifestyle and health hazards. Individual choices and collective interest. In *Health Policy, Ethics and Human Values: European and North American Perspectives* (eds Bunkowski Z, Bryant J H); CIMS, Geneva.

de Vet HCW, van Leeuwen FE (1986). Dietary guidelines for cancer prevention: the etiology of a confused debate. *Nutrition and Cancer* 8: 223–229.

Doll R, Peto R (1981). The causes of cancer. *J Natl Cancer Inst* 66: 1191–1308.

Downie RS (1990). Ethics in Health Education: an introduction. In *Ethics in Health Education* (ed Doxiadis S); J Wiley & Sons Ltd.

Downie RS, Fyfe C, Tannahill A (1990). Health promotion: models and values. Oxford: Oxford University Press.

Doxiadis S (1987). *Ethical dilemmas in Health Promotion*. J Wiley & Sons, Chichester.

Higginson J, Muir CS (1979). Environmental carcinogenesis: misconception and limitations to cancer control. *J Natl Cancer Inst* 63: 1291–1298.

Hill MJ (1988). Cancer prevention. Abstract book of ECP Workshop on "Information and Cancer prevention". Santa Margherita Ligure.

Miettinen OS (1983). Philosophy in a learned profession: observation and thoughts. *Proc R Duch Acad Sci C* 86: 517–523.

National Research Council (1982). Nutrition and Cancer. Washington DC: National Academy Press.

Riis P (1990). Ethics, Health Education and Nutrition. In *Ethics in Health Education* (ed Doxiadis S); J Wilay & Sons Ltd.

Roy D, de Wachter MAM (1988). *Traité d'Anthropologie Médicale*. Cited in Bégin M.

Seedhouse D (1986). *Health: the foundations of achievement*. John Wiley Chichester.

World Health Organization (1946). Constitution. New York.

WHO Health Promotion (1984). A discussion document on the concept and principles. Copenhagen. World Health Education.

Williams G (1984). Health promotion-caring concern or slick salesmanship? *J Med Ethics* **10:** 191–195.

Wynder EL, Gori GB (1977). Contribution of the environment to cancer incidence: an epidemiologic exercise. *J Natl Cancer Inst* **58:** 825–832.

Chapter 17

Risk Assessment: Likely Effect of Dietary Advice on Cancer

HCW DE VET

Department of Epidemiology and Biostatistics
PO Box 616, 6200 MD Maastricht, The Netherlands.

Introduction

In 1985 the European Organization for Cooperation in Cancer Prevention (ECP) and the International Union of Nutritional Sciences (IUNS) held a workshop on diet and human carcinogenesis in Aarhus, Denmark. They issued recommendations to the public, to the food industry, to governments and other organizations and to the scientific community (Consensus statement on provisional dietary guidelines). Meanwhile, further data have become available on different aspects of the prevention of cancer by dietary advice. For this reason, the recommendations of 1985 will be reviewed in the 1991 ECP Symposium.

It is rather shortsighted to formulate an isolated piece of dietary advice directed towards the prevention of only one disease or group of diseases. It goes without saying that only advice that is consistent with good nutritional practice can be given for a specific disease. One dietary factor may have different effects on cancer risk and on the risk of other diseases. It may even have an opposite effect on different types of cancer. For example, dietary fat increases the risk of colon cancer, but probably decreases the risk of stomach cancer (Hill, 1987). In the case of opposite effects on different diseases, the pros and cons have to be weighed against each other. Although it is logical to give dietary advice to improve health in general, this paper directs its attention exclusively to the likely effect of dietary advice on cancer risk. Instead of providing a clear-cut answer on how big the effect of dietary advice is, the paper elaborates on the difficulties that are encountered in assessing the likely effect.

The first part of the paper deals with a theoretical estimation of the likely effect of dietary factors, i.e. the risk assessment. The prominent question in this respect is: how much can the cancer incidence be reduced

175

by a low risk diet and how certain are these data? The second part of the paper concerns the effectiveness of dietary advice in practice. The question here is: are people willing to change their diet for health reasons? Last but not least, the consequences of the uncertainties about the likely effect on the issuing or adaptation of dietary advice are discussed.

Likely effect in theory

Risk assessments

Ten years ago, Doll and Peto published an extensive paper on the causes of cancer (Doll and Peto, 1981). Based on comparisons between cancer mortality in different countries, they estimated that 75–80% of all cancer deaths in the US are avoidable. In these comparisons they correctly excluded countries with unreliable data, but they did not take into account the social acceptability of the required preventive actions. They estimated that 35% of all cancer deaths are attributable to dietary factors. In other words: a low risk diet (whatever that may be) could reduce the cancer mortality by 35%. Doll and Peto's own remark on these estimates was: "It must be emphasised that the figure chosen is highly speculative and chiefly refers to dietary factors which are not yet reliably identified. Experimental findings and human observations alike provide many indications that dietary factors are of major importance in determining the risk of cancers of the gastrointestinal tract, some cancers of the female sex organs, and epithelial cancers in general, but there is as yet little decisive evidence on which firm conclusions can be based". The uncertainty is underlined by the broad margins of their estimate, with a lower limit of 10% and an upper limit of 70%.

A more precise way to estimate the role of diet in cancer prevention is by calculation of the population-attributable-risk proportion (PAR). The PAR for a binary exposure is defined as $P_e(RR-1)/(P_e(RR-1)+1)$, where RR is the risk ratio for the exposure category, with the non-exposed as reference, and P_e is the proportion of the population in the exposed category (Rothman, 1986). However, dietary exposures are not simply dichotomous. Usually a measurement on a continuous or interval scale is categorized in 3, 4 or more categories. The PAR can be calculated if the risk ratio for each category and the proportion of the population in each category is known. The preventable proportion can be calculated from the PARs if the shift in proportions of the population over the various categories by dietary change is known (Wahrendorf, 1987). In this way, an estimation of the reduction in cancer incidence was made, based on some case-control studies on colon and stomach cancer (Wahrendorf, 1987). The preventable proportion was calculated under two different assumptions: firstly that 100% of the population from each category above the lowest risk category would shift to the next one down, and secondly under the more realistic assumption that 50% of the population could be persuaded to do so. A shift of 50% of the population to a lower risk diet was estimated to reduce the incidence of colon and stomach cancer by 15–20%.

Another example of such an approach was published recently, concerning the effect of dietary factors on breast cancer (Howe *et al.*, 1990). In a combined analysis of 12 case-control studies the intake of fat and vitamin C appeared to influence breast cancer risk. Based on the estimates of the risk ratios for the various exposure categories, the preventable proportion was calculated. A 16% reduction in breast cancer incidence for premenopausal women and a 24% reduction for postmenopausal women was predicted, if all women reduced their saturated fat intake to 9% of their total caloric intake and increased their vegetable and fruit consumption to reach a daily vitamin C intake of 380 mg (which is quite high). However, these calculations are dependent on the validity of the data, the causality of the associations, and the achievable level of dietary changes.

It is important to note at this point that the PARs of all risk factors of a specific cancer do not need to count up to 100%. Carcinogenesis is considered to be a multi-stage process, and every stage is influenced by various factors. Only if all necessary factors are present can cancer occur. This means that the occurrence of cancer may be attributed to every necessary factor in the chain of causation. Thus the sum of the PARs may be much larger than 100% (Rothman, 1986).

Evidence from Non-experimental Studies

The results of a study are valid if the study is free of bias. A case-control design, which is the most frequently used in the diet-cancer area, is especially susceptible to bias. Bias may occur due to imperfect recall of the study subjects of their dietary intake. Moreover, cases and controls may give different reports of their food consumption, e.g. because cases are influenced by their disease status or because interviewers approach cases and controls differently. This leads to differential recall bias. For the sake of convenience and to reduce recall bias, dietary information is usually obtained with regard to the period just before diagnosis of the disease, either presuming that this is the aetiologically relevant moment, or presuming that current food habits reflect food habits in the past. In the latter case, the reliability of the information depends on the extent to which recent food intake is associated with the intake in the aetiologically relevant period. (Carcinogenesis is considered to be a long lasting multi-stage process. The timing of the aetiologically relevant period depends on whether a factor is active in an early or later phase of the cancer process).

A comparable degree of imprecise recall in cases and controls leads to underestimation of the effect, whereas differential recall bias in cases and controls may lead to either underestimation and overestimation of the effect (Rothman, 1986).

In cohort studies, recall bias is less of a problem, since information about dietary habits is obtained long before the diagnosis of cancer. However, the above mentioned problems with respect to collecting precise and aetiologically relevant information about the intake of dietary factors, occur to the same extent as in case-control studies. However, in cohort studies with repeated measurements of the food consumption (Brandt *et al.*, 1990), the stability of the food intake can be examined. Moreover, if the cohort study starts with a rather young population, even the timing of the aetiologically relevant period could be assessed. Another advantage of cohort studies compared to case-control studies is that the effect of dietary factors can be studied on the incidence of all types of cancers and all other diseases. This enables us to judge the effect on health in general.

An issue that plagues both case-control and cohort studies is confounding bias. A confounding factor is a factor that is both associated with the presumed risk factor and with the disease under study. Theoretically, if not prevented by the study design, confounding can be adjusted for in the analysis. In practice this is only true for confounding factors that are known and properly measured. Confounding bias may cause either underestimation or overestimation of the effect. In dietary studies confounding is almost always present. If the data are analysed on the nutrient level, confounding is present because some nutrients mainly occur in the same foods. For example, persons with a high vegetable and fruit consumption will show a high dietary intake of beta-carotene as well as a high intake of vitamin C and dietary fibre. This evokes the question as to which of these factors is the causal agent, in other words, which factor is responsible for the cancer preventive effect. Risk factors that do not have a causal relationship with the disease, but which are associated with it, are sometimes called risk indicators. It is important to note that intervention on these risk indicators does not exert any effect on the prevention of cancer. With respect to the energy containing nutrients, people with a high fat intake (expressed as a percentage of caloric intake) have, by definition, a lower percentage of their energy from carbohydrates. Mutatis mutandis, if the analysis is on the food product level, special combinations of products, usually eaten together, are highly correlated and this again may lead to confounding bias. For that reason, analyses of food patterns, without pointing to specific dietary factors, should be promoted. Note that dietary advice is always given on the level of food products or food patterns. The suboptimal validity of non-experimental studies seriously hampers the estimation of the likely effect of dietary intervention, and mainly for the following reasons:

1. The risk estimation in non-experimental studies may be precarious. On the one hand, because of possible differential recall bias (especially in case-control studies) and because of confounding due to improper adjustment, the risk ratio's found may be either over- or underestimated. With the weak associations that are usually observed, it is difficult to judge whether there is an effect or not. On the other hand, because of imprecise information, which always lead to an underestimation of the effect, the risk ratios may be more pronounced than found in most studies. Thus, the effect may not be present at all, or may be much larger than suggested by the risk ratio. This calls for a broad range of uncertainty around the estimation of the likely effect.

2. A factor A found to be associated with cancer incidence may be a risk indicator. In fact, another factor B is responsible for the effect. This is very easily visualized in the case of nutrients that mainly occur in the same foods. Dietary intervention on factor A would not then necessarily affect cancer incidence; it would do so only if the intake of factor B is also influenced by the intervention on factor A. This may or may not be the case. Whether a factor has causal influence can only be assessed in an experimental study.

3. A factor may have an effect on cancer incidence but only in an early phase of the cancer process. The effect may be found in non-experimental studies because, in case of rather stable dietary intake, recent intake may reflect intake in the far past. But this does not imply that changes of intake influence cancer incidence in the short run. If the aetiologically relevant period is in an early phase of the process, only an early start of a low risk diet may reduce cancer.

Because of the above mentioned factors, on the basis of non-experimental studies only rough estimation can be provided about the likely effect of dietary factors. In other words, the effect of dietary intervention on cancer incidence is not guaranteed by findings in non-experimental studies.

Evidence from Experimental Studies

The first thing to say is that experimental studies are not a panacea for all the problems encountered in non-experimental studies. Some problems are solved, but others arise. The experimental studies on diet and cancer have as their main advantage over non-experimental studies, that the problems of confounding bias can be avoided by randomization (Roth-man, 1986). The new problems mostly have to do with feasibility and the need to make more explicit choices in the study design. The study population of the trials should be large, as the incidence of cancer is very low. If the trials are restricted to a certain phase of the cancer process, by making use of biomarkers, the study population may be somewhat smaller and more pronounced effects may be observed, since the relations studied are more specific (Lippman *et al*, 1990). In general, choices have to be made on the intervention (which food factor in which dose, or which dietary modifications should be advised), on the study population (age, sex, high risk groups), on the duration of the trial, and on the outcome parameter. The intervention is only effective if the aetiologically relevant period is involved. If this is not the case, a non-experimental study will show an effect only to the extent that the food intake during the aetiologically relevant period is associated with the assessed food intake, while a trial will show no effect at all.

Two types of experiments can be distinguished: trials in which the effect of an isolated food factor (usually a micronutrient) is examined, and experiments which assess the effect of dietary modification. In the latter case, the dietary changes are brought about by dietary advice.

In experiments on isolated food factors the factors may be administered as supplements in a double-blind design. These trials have a high validity, but on the other hand their application is limited: only trials and dietary factors with presumably favourable effects on cancer incidence are ethically justified. The choice of which dietary factor should be tested is crucial. For example, based on the finding in non-experimental studies that a high consumption of vegetables is inversely associated with cancer incidence, the dietary factors beta-carotene, vitamin C, dietary fibre, indoles etc (or special combinations of these factors) may be chosen. But if the choice is wrong, i.e. a risk indicator is tested, no effect at all will be observed. On the other hand, if an effect is found, there is convincing evidence that this factor has a causal relationship with cancer incidence. In these trials with an isolated food factor, the extrapolation of the observed effect to the impact on cancer incidence by dietary modification, i.e. influencing the same nutritional factor under more natural conditions, remains to be made. It has to be noted in this respect that the dose of dietary factors in such trials is many-fold the average daily intake, and can hardly be reached by diet alone. This hampers the direct translation of these results to the likely effect of dietary advice.

In experimental studies on the effect of dietary modifications, half of the population should be advised to modify their dietary habits on some points, while the other half of the population goes without advice. The study population cannot be blinded in that case. Therefore it is possible that the part of the population who did not receive the dietary advice, also change their food habits in the presumed favourable direction. This will dilute the contrast between the experimental and control group and possibly mask a potential effect. This diluting effect occurred for example in the Multiple Risk Factor Intervention Trial (MRFIT), a large trial which was aimed at assessing the effect of intervention on risk factors for coronary heart disease (MRFIT Research Group, 1982). In addition, poor compliance with the dietary advice by the study population may further decrease the contrast between the experimental and control group. As opposed to trials with an isolated food factor, a specific hypothesis (on exactly which factor is responsible for the effect on cancer) is not necessary: it is possible to test the effect of a 'low risk' food pattern. As long as the factors responsible for the cancer preventive effect are indeed modified, a potential effect will be observed. From these studies the translation to the likely effect of dietary advice in practice is easier to make than in trials with an isolated food factor. Actually, the trial does not test the effect of the specific dietary modification, but the effect of the advice to modify the diet, thus taking non-compliance into account. In fact, the compliance of the study population might be even better than the compliance of the public in practice.

At this moment several trials on isolated food factors (mainly beta-carotene and vitamin C) are under way (Dewys *et al.*, 1986). Some trials with high risk populations, or populations with a precancerous lesion have been published (Greenberg *et al.*, 1990; Vet *et al.*, 1991; Stich *et al.*, 1988; McKeown-Eyssen *et al.*, 1988; Munoz *et al.*, 1987). The results are less promising than expected. The results of ongoing trials are eagerly awaited.

In some large trials on risk factor intervention for cardiovascular disease, data are available on the effect on cancer risk (Coleman and Law, 1990). The risk factors intervened on were smoking, cholesterol, blood pressure and sometimes physical activity. The advised diet was low fat, or saturated fat partly replaced by unsaturated fat. In a few trials the expected reduction in cancer incidence or mortality was observed (e.g. on lung cancer risk) but in others no effect on cancer risk was found, and in some trials the frequency of cancer increased. As the intervention was on all risk factors simultaneously, the effect of dietary advice cannot be isolated in these trials. The effects found on cancer risk are rather disappointing. However, it has to be noted that the numbers of cancer cases in these trials were small, the intervention was not especially directed at cancer prevention, and the period of follow-up might have been too short to observe an effect on cancer incidence or mortality.

In the near future, more information about the relationship between diet and cancer will become available, but we should not be too optimistic. Well performed cohort studies may provide further evidence on the risk estimates, either changing the point estimate or narrowing the range of uncertainty. However, the problems of confounding bias remain. These problems may be circumvented by the experimental design. The randomized studies with isolated food factors have produced some interesting results so far, and probably will do so in the near future. Experiences with the trials on risk factor intervention with respect to cardiovascular diseases do not motivate researchers to start large intervention studies on the effect of dietary modification on cancer risk. An intervention study on dietary fat to reduce breast cancer risk has been proposed (Prentice *et al.*, 1988). However, problems with reaching enough contrast in fat intake between the experimental and control group and recent data on the fat-breast cancer issue tempers the enthusiasm to some extent (Greenwald, 1988). As far as I know, no other intervention studies for cancer prevention by dietary modification are planned. This means that the theoretical risk estimation will keep its large range of uncertainty for the present.

Likely Effect in Practice

People cannot be manipulated like laboratory rats, with respect to food habits. Laboratory rats just consume the food that is offered; most people are free to choose their own diet. Their dietary behaviour is influenced by several factors, and health considerations may be one of these. Before answering the question on how dietary advice affects dietary behaviour, a health education model is presented that categorizes the various factors that determine health behaviour in general. This model is an adaptation of the Fishbein-Ajzen model (Ajzen and Fishbein, 1980). It states that external factors influence behaviour along three different pathways: attitude, subjective norms, and self-efficacy (Vries *et al.*, 1988).

Attitude refers to the knowledge and beliefs of a person concerning the specific consequences of a certain form of behaviour. An attitude is the weighing (both consciously and unconsciously) of all the advantages and disadvantages of performance of the behaviour, as seen by the individual. Health is only one of the possible considerations, and is often a relatively unimportant one.

Subjective norm is a concept that refers to the influence of others; directly by what others expect, indirectly by what others do (modelling). The influence of subjective norm is dependent on whether a person is inclined to agree with opinions of others.

Self-efficacy stands for the perceived capacity to be able to conform to the (desirable) behaviour. It involves an estimation of ability, taking into account possible internal or external barriers (e.g. internal: insufficient knowledge, skill or endurance etc; external: resistance from others, time or money not available, conflicting life-style etc).

After this theoretical excursion I will discuss how dietary advice may influence dietary behaviour.

Self-efficacy is very important in the case of dietary change in order to influence cancer risk. As the potential benefits will be encountered only after a long time, the persons have to change their habits permanently, and not only temporarily. This surely influences the perceived perception of ability to perform such a life-time behaviour.

The *subjective norm* with respect to dietary behaviour will only change slowly on the basis of dietary advice. For example, in the case of smoking behaviour, it has taken a long time before smoking became disapproved of by public opinion. Disapproval of unhealthy food habits may possibly increase in the future.

Dietary advice supposedly has most influence on dietary behaviour via a change of attitude. Dietary advice will inform people about dietary factors that affect cancer risk. It will give information that will help them in weighing pros and cons of certain behaviour. Consequently, their beliefs about the positive and negative consequences of their behaviour would possibly change. However, it is difficult for people to make a realistic risk interpretation. The estimation of the potential advantages of dietary change is complicated by at least three factors:

–   Firstly, the risk estimations show a wide range of uncertainty. In the education of the public, this uncertainty hampers the provision of clear figures about the impact on cancer. Therefore, it is difficult (if not impossible) for people to perceive realistically the potential advantages of dietary changes.

–   Secondly, the relation between dietary factors and cancer is not readily visible to the population. For example, it is not as clear as is the relation between smoking and lung cancer. Although many smokers do not contract lung cancer, the majority of people who do get lung cancer are indeed smokers. People who contract, for example, cancer of the stomach or colon do not have a visibly unhealthier diet than persons who remain free of these cancers.

–   Thirdly, the potential benefits do not follow immediately. The expected reward for the dietary change may only be encountered after a very long time. This surely does not motivate people to maintain dietary changes.

For these reasons, health arguments may be judged to be not as important as health professionals would want them to be. Besides, several other factors influence dietary behaviour, most of them yielding immediate rewards.

As a starting point, the cultural background determines the basic food habits of a person. Even between European countries the food habits differ: the Scandinavian countries have different food habits than are seen in the Mediterranean areas. Some food habits are very difficult to change because they are based on cultural values and beliefs that are deeply rooted in people's life (Rosin and Vollmecke, 1986). Gastronomical aspects play an important role. People choose foods that they like because of sensorial characteristics, such as taste, appearance, consistency. Economical reasons may be involved. Especially for poor people, prices of food may be an important factor. On the other hand, sometimes expensive foods are preferred in order to give expression to standing, for example when other people are invited round or when there is a party. Convenience reasons may also play a role. People may prefer foods that are quick and easy to prepare (fast foods) in order to keep more time for other activities.

In conclusion, dietary behaviour is not easy to influence, and knowledge abut risk factors will play only a minor role in this process (Axelson *et al.*, 1985). According to health educators, a more integral approach will enhance the compliance to dietary advice (Leeuw, 1989). Such a health promotion approach includes, besides health education, facilitating and regulatory activities, e.g. making unhealthy foods more expensive, increasing the supply of healthy foods in shops and canteens, or producing substitutes such as artificial sweeteners and low-fat products. An example in the diet-cancer field of such a health promotion programme is the Cancer and Diet Intervention Project in Minnesota (Potter *et al.*, 1990).

Risk Assessment and Dietary Advice

As was already announced in the introduction, this paper does not provide clear-cut answers about the effect of dietary advice. The risk assessments based on the available evidence still show a broad range of uncertainty. This implies that the likely effect of dietary advice is difficult to predict. Another uncertain factor is the compliance of the public to dietary advice. This makes statements about the likely effect of dietary advice which are even more precarious. What are the consequences of these uncertainties for the issuing of dietary advice? Should dietary advice be postponed until more firm evidence is available? And if so, when is the evidence strong enough? There are a couple of sound and less sound arguments in favour of issuing dietary advice on scanty evidence on the likely effects. The argument that is often used is that, although the benefits are not exactly known, they will surely outweigh the disadvantages. This might be true, but it ignores disadvantages such as the cost and the efforts for the people to change their diet. Moreover the diet may arouse feelings of frustration and guilt. First, this holds for healthy individuals trying hard, but in vain, to conform to the dietary advice. Second, adherers to the advice may feel very frustrated if they still contract cancer. And finally, cancer patients who were not willing or able to comply with the advice may feel very guilty.

Another argument for issuing advice despite rather poor evidence is that the public is exposed to all kinds of messages on diet and cancer. Findings of various types of research (e.g. animal and laboratory studies, remarkable findings in single case-control studies) are reported in the newspapers. It is very difficult, if not impossible, for lay people to estimate the importance of these messages. Dietary advice issued by official committees may function as a counterbalance for this uncontrolled information. It is also often argued that dietary advice for cancer prevention is justified, because it is consistent with good nutritional practice. This argument is somewhat remarkable. If the dietary advice for cancer prevention does not deviate from the dietary guidelines for health in general, special advice for cancer prevention is not necessary. But if it does deviate, this argument does not apply.

The discussion about dietary advice based on rather poor evidence on likely effects took place almost a decade ago, when several committees considered issuing dietary recommendations for cancer prevention (Council for Agriculture Science and Technology; Vet and Leeuwen, 1986). Now it is time to discuss the necessity of adapting this advice based on current knowledge. In my opinion, the evidence required for changing or detailing dietary advice is far stronger than for issuing the first guidelines. This opinion is based on two arguments:

–   Dietary advice should be as simple and unequivocal as possible. If the advice is too detailed, it is more difficult for the people to recall the information. For example, the advice to eat more vegetables, but not the vegetables with a high nitrate content, is very confusing for the public. This is only wise to do, if the effects on health will compensate the lower compliance because of the difficulty of the message. The evidence for detailed information should be stronger than the evidence for broad advice. Moreover, dietary advice for specific cancer prevention, that has no positive effect on other diseases, should be considered with more caution.

–   Contradiction of previous advice should be avoided at all times, because this frustrates the public: people won't believe anything afterwards. That is another reason why the advice should only be further detailed if it is justified by very strong evidence. The chance that advice has to be changed later must be minimised.

Conclusion

The likely effect of dietary advice on cancer prevention is surrounded by uncertainties. Current knowledge does not prompt adaptation of the dietary advice given by the ECP in 1985. Future research may lessen the range of uncertainty around the risk estimates, thereby providing a more firm basis for health education and promotion.

References

Ajzen I, Fishbein M (1980). Understanding attitudes and predicting social behaviour. Prentice Hall, Englewood Cliffs, NJ, USA.

Axelson ML, Federline TO, Brinberg D (1985). A meta-analysis of food- and nutrition-related research. *J Nutr Educ* **17:** 51–4.

Brandt PA van den, Goldbohm RA, Veer P van't, Volovics A, Hermus RJJ, Sturmans F (1990). A large-scale prospective study on diet and cancer in the Netherlands. *J Clin Epidemiol* **43:** 285–95.

Coleman MP, Law M (1990). Prevention of cancer: review of the evidence from intervention trials. In: Evaluating effectiveness of primary prevention of cancer. Eds Hakama M, Beral V, Cullen J W, Parkin D M. IARC Scientific Publications No 103, International Agency for Research on Cancer.

Consensus statement on provisional dietary guidelines (1985). Joint ECP-IUNS Workshop on Diet and Human Carcinogenesis. In: Diet and Human Carcinogenesis, Proceedings of the 3rd Annual Symposium of the European Organization for Cooperation in Cancer Prevention Studies (ECP), Aahrus, Denmark, June 19–21. Eds J V Joossens, M J Hill, J Geboers. International Congress Series 685. Excerpta Medica, Amsterdam.

Council for Agriculture Science and Technology (1982). Diet, nutrition and cancer: a critique. Special Publication No 13.

Dewys WD, Malone WF, Butrum RR, Sestili MA (1986). Clinical trial in cancer prevention. *Cancer* (Suppl) **58:** 1954–62.

Doll R, Peto R (1981). The causes of cancer. *J Natl Cancer Inst* **66:** 1191–1308.

Greenwald P (1988). Issues raised by the Women's Health Trial. *J Natl Cancer Inst* **80:** 788–90.

Greenberg ER, Baron JA, Stukel TA, Stevens MM, Mandel JS *et al.* (1990). A clinical trial of beta-catotene to prevent basal-cell and squamous cell cancers of the skin. *N Engl J Med* **323:** 789–95.

Hill MJ (1987). Dietary fat and human cancer. *Anticancer Res* **7:** 281–92.

Howe GR, Hirohata T, Hislop TG, Iscovich JM, Yuan J-M *et al.* (1990). Dietary factors and risk of breast cancer. Combined analysis of 12 case-control studies. *J Natl Cancer Inst* **82:** 561-9.

Leeuw E de (1989). The sane revolution; health promotion. Assen, The Netherlands. Van Gorkum.

Lippman SM, Lee JS, Lotan R, Hittelman W, Wargovich MJ, Hong WK (1990). Biomarkers as intermediate end points in chemoprevention trials. *J Natl Cancer Inst* **82:** 555–560.

McKeown-Eyssen G, Holloway C, Jazmaji V, Bright-See E, Dion P, Bruce WR (1988). A randomized trial of vitamin C and E in the prevention of recurrence of colorectal polyps. *Cancer Res* **48**: 4701–5.

MRFIT Research Group (1982). Multiple Risk Factor Intervention trial: Risk factor changes and mortality results. *JAMA* **248**: 1465-77.

Munoz N, Hayashi M, Lu J-B, Wahrendorf J, Crespi M, Bosch FX (1987). The effect of riboflavin, retinol and zinc on micronuclei of buccal mucosa and of oesophagus: A randomized double-blind intervention study in China. *J Natl Cancer Inst* **79**: 687–91.

Potter JD, Graves KL, Finnegan JR, Mullis RM, Baxter JS *et al.* (1990). The cancer and diet intervention project to reduce nutrition-related risk of cancer. *Health Educ Res* **5**: 489–503.

Prentice RL, Kakar F, Hursting S, Sheppard L, Klein R, Kushi LH (1988). Aspects of the rationale for the Women's Health Trial. *J Natl Cancer Inst* **80**: 802–13.

Rosin P, Vollmecke TA (1986). Food likes and dislikes. *Ann Rev Nutr* **6**: 433–456.

Rothman KJ (1986). Modern Epidemiology. Little, Brown and Company, Boston.

Stich HF, Rosin MP, Hornby AP, Mathew B, Sankaranarayanan S, Nair K (1988). Remission of oral leukoplakias and micronuclei in tobacco/betel quid chewers treated with beta-carotene and with beta-carotene plus vitamin A. *Int J Cancer* **42**: 195–9.

Vet HCW de, Leeuwen FE van (1986). Dietary guidelines for cancer prevention: the etiology of a confused debate. *Nutr Cancer* **8**: 223–9.

Vet HCW de, Knipschild PG, Willebrand D, Schouten HJA, Sturmans F (1991). The effect of beta-carotene on the regression and progression of cervical dysplasia: a clinical experiment. *J Clin Epidemiol* **44**: 273–83.

Vries H de, Dijkstra M, Kuhlman P (1988). Self-efficacy: the third factor besides attitude and subjective norm as a predictor of behavioural intentions. *Health Educ Res* **3**: 273–82.

Wahrendorf J (1987). An estimate of the proportion of colo-rectal and stomach cancer which might be prevented by certain changes in dietary habits. *Int J Cancer* **40**: 625–8.

CHAPTER 18

Final Conclusions

MJ HILL, E BENITO, A GIACOSA

During the last two decades many groups have attempted to summarize the current knowledge on diet and cancer and to present the conclusions in the form of sets of guidelines. These have been reviewed here in the symposium. For example, in 1985 ECP and IUNS organized a joint workshop on diet and cancer which produced just such a set of guidelines. Since then much has happened in the field of diet and cancer and so it was decided that it would be timely to update those guidelines. Here we present the conclusions from the workshop held in parallel with the symposium (as described in the Foreword).

There was a lack of consensus amongst the experts on modification of the 1985 guidelines because of the important differences observed in the results of recent epidemiological studies carried out in different countries. It was concluded from this that the evidence is not sufficiently strong or coherent to make recommendations for the population in general, although guidelines targeted at specific populations could be justified. In addition, whereas the ECP-IUNS (and most other) guidelines were drafted in terms of nutrients, the evidence for these is weak but is very much stronger for food groups.

The presentation of general guidelines to the world in general always appeared to be a gross oversimplification and in our current state of knowledge is now impossible to justify. For example, in North America and Australia a high fat diet is associated with a high risk of colorectal and of breast cancer as well as of ischaemic heart disease (IHD); in consequence many European groups have issued guidelines recommending a decrease in fat consumption for European countries in general. However, it was reported in the symposium that in many parts of the Mediterranean region the intake of fat is higher than it is in the northern countries; since they do not have the expected high risk of the cancers or of IHD why should they change their diet? and why should we make guidelines that imply that they should change to a low fat diet? Similarly, most sets of guidelines recommend an increased intake of dietary fibre to prevent colorectal and breast cancers; however, we now know that the scientific basis of this guideline cannot be substantiated. Since it is now recognized that an unknown proportion of the dietary starch intake reaches the colon and there behaves as non-starch polysaccharide (i.e. dietary fibre), the physiological basis for the definitions and the assays of dietary fibre must be reassessed. Despite these new problems in assessing the role of these nutrients in human carcinogenesis, the raw data from case-control epidemiological studies in terms of foods and food groups remains valid.

Two of the usual epidemiological observations have been strengthened by more recent data. The first is that a low intake of fresh vegetables and fruit is associated with a high risk of cancer at a number of sites (e.g. the stomach, colorectum, breast, endometrium, ovary). The reasons for this in terms of vitamins and micronutrients, trace elements, dietary fibre, phytate, anticarcinogens etc are not clear but, if we elect to concentrate on food groups, need not be important. Similarly, a low intake of cereals is associated with a high risk of colorectal cancer in the northern but less strongly in the southern countries of Europe. This, too cannot be explained in terms of the nutrients but this need not be important if we restrict our discussion to food groups.

The second is the strong association between obesity and risk of cancer at a number of sites. Since obesity is associated with a number of prominent non-malignant diseases (such as diabetes, IHD, blood pressure) the control of obesity should be one of the major public health targets in all European countries. Obesity is the result of excess energy intake over expenditure, and so can be controlled by decreased energy intake or by increased exercise or both. There is no evidence that either of these *per se* influence cancer risk except through their effect on body weight. In consequence there is no reason from human studies to recommend a low energy intake if the person is not overweight.

Our problems with regard to dietary fat have already been mentioned but need to be considered in more detail. Our 1985 guideline, like that of most groups, was to decrease fat intake from the current figure of more than 40% of calories to less than 30%. This was based largely on human data from North America and Australia supported by results from animal studies. However, the recent results from European case-control studies do not implicate fat in colorectal or breast carcinogenesis as strongly as did the previous non-European studies. Furthermore, populations in southern Europe with low incidences of the "fat-related" cancers often have higher fat intakes than do the northern populations with their high risks of the relevant cancers. Clearly the situation is not as clear as it appeared in 1985 and the dietary guideline proposed at that time for Europe cannot be substantiated for the southern half of the continent. In addition some populations in northern Europe have been recommended to abandon the frying pan in favour of cooking methods which decrease the fat content of the food. In many parts of Spain and Portugal frying is the most popular cooking method; since they have low incidences of the "fat-related" cancers why should they change their cooking methods? It is clear that any guidelines on dietary fat must be closely targeted at high-risk groups rather than at the population of Europe. The best evidence from northern Europe still indicates an association between animal fat intake and risk of cancer of the colorectum, breast, endometrium ovary and prostate (as well as IHD); in consequence advice to decrease the amount of dietary meat and dairy products remains valid when targeted to northern European populations. The low risk of the "fat-related" cancers and IHD in the Mediterranean areas is strong evidence that these areas should not abandon their traditional diet, since the favoured alternative of a "hamburger fast-food" diet rich in animal fat is likely to carry a health penalty.

The area of greatest change since 1985 is that of dietary fibre. Advice given, particularly to northern European populations, to increase their intake of dietary fibre in order to decrease the risk of a number of digestive tract diseases (including colorectal cancer) as well as breast cancer, IHD, diabetes etc. now looks far from firmly based. A British Nutrition Foundation Task Force (BNF, 1990) on complex carbohydrates in foods concluded that "hypotheses that many 'western' diseases such as colonic diverticulosis, colorectal cancer and irritable bowel syndrome are caused by a deficiency of 'dietary fibre' have not been substantiated; nor have hypotheses that fibre can protect against diabetes, obesity and coronary heart disease". A major source of confusion has been the failure to realize until recently that a variable proportion of dietary starch is not digested in the small bowel and so enters the large bowel where it behaves as non-starch polysaccharide. At our present state of knowledge we cannot predict how much starch escapes digestion in this way, because it depends on the length and temperature of cooking and the temperature at which it is consumed. However, we can be certain that it normally greatly exceeds the amount of "dietary fibre" entering the colon. In consequence all epidemiological studies of dietary fibre and disease (e.g. case control studies of "dietary fibre" and colorectal cancer) must be reassessed. However, the raw data on food groups from which the (erroneous) calculations of colonic carbohydrate were made remain valid. The recommendation to populations in northern Europe to increase their intake of cereals (their main source of non-starch polysaccharide) and of potatoes (a major source of colonic starch) is valid, although the case-control studies carried out in the Mediterranean countries (where the main cereal is rice) are much less convincing and no guideline on cereal consumption can be made.

In the discussion on meat and protein it was concluded that there was no evidence that the protein component of meat was a risk factor for the "diseases of affluence"; the risks associated with meat consumption (e.g. in the cohort studies of nurses in relation to cancer of the colon and breast) are related to the fat component and not to the protein in meat. In consequence the recommendations to remove the visible fat from red meat, to substitute poultry for red meat, and also to cook in ways that decrease (e.g. grilling) rather than increase (e.g. frying) the fat content remain valid for those populations where the fat consumption appears to be a risk factor. In support of this, the cohort study of nurses showed that for colon cancer red meat was a greater risk factor than poultry.

In addition to containing carcinogens/mutagens many foods also contain anticarcinogens, including the antioxidant vitamins (A, C and E) and the provitamin carotene. However, whilst there is strong evidence that foods rich in these compounds are associated with a low risk of many of the most common cancers, there is little clear evidence of the identity of the protective agents. In consequence, once again, we must conclude that the justification for guidelines is stronger for foods and food groups than it is for nutrients or micronutrients.

Finally, it is necessary to address the problem of food additives since these compounds receive more attention in the media than all of the rest of the diet. It must be reiterated that there is no evidence that these compounds make any significant contribution to our cancer risk. In consequence, where the additives protect the nutritional quality of the food (e.g. antimicrobial compounds, antioxidants which prevent rancidity of fat etc) there is every reason to continue their use. The health hazards associated with food spoilage are acute and well understood, and greatly outweigh possible long-term risks and so the risk-benefit balance is clear. Where the additive has no nutrient value and does not protect the food against spoilage etc. the risk-benefit analysis is less simple; the possible small risk of cancer is not offset by any health benefit but only an organoleptic one, and the risk is more difficult to defend.

The preceding conclusions present the basis on which guidelines could be formulated. These need to be in two components – the basic guidelines and the means by which they can be applied to a specific target population. The workshop participants considered that there were major gaps in our knowledge of public health education techniques, and that there is much work to be done in developing tools for educating and motivating the public. What is clear is that the adaptation of the guidelines and their application to a specific population should be carried out by local or national organizations and could not be done centrally. The important differences in food consumption patterns in different European countries and the need to disseminate the information throughout the public education information network were major arguments in favour of this.

In consequence, these conclusions should be taken as guidelines to be elaborated by both the government institutions and the National Leagues against Cancer in each European country for application to the specific national or local situation.

Index of Authors

Index

additives, food, 192
adenocarcinomas, renal cell, 93
adenomas, large bowel, 60–1
advice, dietary, *see* recommendations
age of tissue, cancer risk related to, 37
alcohol (ethanol), 20, 59–60, 115–29, *see also specific types of alcoholic beverage*
    large bowel cancer and, 59–60, 61
    in Mediterranean countries, availability/consumption, 136, 137
    oral cavity/pharyngeal/oesophageal cancers and, 116–25
    reduced consumption, recommended, 22
    tobacco and, joint effects, 116–19, 125
alimentary tract, *see specific areas*
amines, aromatic, 15, 79
    food processing producing, 79
animal fat in Mediterranean countries, availability/consumption, 136, 137, 140
animal studies, assessing value, 43–50
anticarcinogens (inhibitors of carcinogenesis), 21, 25–33, 192, *see also specific anticarcinogens*
    mechanisms of action, 25–6, 26–8
antioxidants, 27
    gastric cancer and, 81
apple cider and apple jack, oesophageal cancer and, 123–4
aromatic amines, *see* amines
arsenic, 15
ascorbic acid, *see* vitamin C
attitude, dietary behaviour and effects of, 182
azoxymethane-initiated tumours, 30, 45

bacterial fermentation of fibre in colon, 87
beer
    oral cavity/pharyngeal/oesophageal cancer and, 117, 122, 123
    rectal cancer and, 59–60
behaviour, dietary, external factors influencing, 182–3

benzene, 16
beta-carotene, *see* β-carotene
bias
    confounding, 178
    recall, 177–8
bile acids, colorectal tumours and, 60–1
bowel, large, *see entries under* intestinal; intestine
bran, anticarcinogenicity, 56
breast
    atypical lobules in, 70
    cancer, 69–73, 92, 93, 94, 103–5
        fat and, 103–5
        in Mediterranean countries, rates, 138, 139–41
        protective factors, 30
        weight and, 71, 92, 93, 94
butyrate, anti-neoplastic action, 29

calcium, large bowel cancer and, 58–9
caloric intake, 18–20, 91–2
    breast cancer and, 69
    high, *see* overnutrition
    large bowel adenomas and, 60
Canada, Department of National Health and Welfare of, Nutrition Recommendations, 9–10
canning of fish in various oils, 158
carbohydrate, carcinogenic potency, 18–19
carcinogens, dietary, 13–24, *see also* precarcinogens
    inhibitors, *see* anticarcinogens
    mutagenic, 15–18
    scavenging/inactivation, 27, 29–30
    transport, inhibition, 27
cardiovascular disease, 144, *see also* coronary heart disease
carotene(s), 39
    gastric cancer and, 80
β-carotene (provitamin A), 39, 40
    gastric cancer and, 80
    large bowel cancer and, 57
cereals

194